MEDICAL AUTHORITY AND ENGLISHWOMEN'S HERBAL TEXTS, 1550–1650

Literary and Scientific Cultures of Early Modernity

Series editors:

This series provides a forum for groundbreaking work on the relations between literary and scientific discourses in Europe, during a period when both fields were in a crucial moment of historical formation. We welcome proposals for books that address the many overlaps between modes of imaginative writing typical of the sixteenth and seventeenth centuries – poetics, rhetoric, prose narrative, dramatic production, utopia – and the vocabularies, conceptual models, and intellectual methods of newly emergent "scientific" fields such as medicine, astronomy, astrology, alchemy, psychology, mapping, mathematics, or natural history. In order to reflect the nature of intellectual inquiry during the period, the series is interdisciplinary in orientation and publishes monographs, edited collections, and selected critical editions of primary texts relevant to an understanding of the mutual implication of literary and scientific epistemologies.

Other titles in the series:

Psychosomatic Disorders in Seventeenth-Century French Literature
Bernadette Höfer

Of Books and Botany in Early Modern England
Sixteenth-Century Plants and Print Culture
Leah Knight

Milton's Secrecy
And Philosophical Hermeneutics
James Dougal Fleming

Biblical Scholarship, Science and Politics in Early Modern England
Thomas Browne and the Thorny Place of Knowledge
Kevin Killeen

Medical Authority and Englishwomen's Herbal Texts, 1550–1650

REBECCA LAROCHE
University of Colorado at Colorado Springs, USA

ASHGATE

Published by
Ashgate Publishing Limited
Wey Court East
Union Road
Farnham
Surrey, GU9 7PT
England

Ashgate Publishing Company
Suite 420
101 Cherry Street
Burlington
VT 05401-4405
USA

www.ashgate.com

British Library Cataloguing in Publication Data
Laroche, Rebecca.
Medical Authority and Englishwomen's Herbal Texts, 1550–1650. – (Literary and Scientific Cultures of Early Modernity)
1. Herbals – England – Early works to 1800. 2. Medical writing – History – 16th century. 3. Medical writing – History –17th century. 4. Literature and medicine – England – History – 16th century. 5. Literature and medicine – England – History – 17th century. 6. Women and literature – England – History – 16th century. 7. Women and literature – England – History – 17th century.
I. Title II. Series
820.9'3561'09031–dc22

Library of Congress Cataloging-in-Publication Data
Laroche, Rebecca.
Medical Authority and Englishwomen's herbal texts, 1550–1650 / by Rebecca Laroche.
p. cm. -- (Literary and Scientific Cultures of Early Modernity)
Includes bibliographical references and index.
1. English prose literature – Women authors – History and criticism. 2. English prose literature – Early modern, 1500–1700 – History and criticism. 3. Herbals – Great Britain – History. 4. Literature and medicine – Great Britain – History – 16th century. 5. Literature and medicine – Great Britain – History – 17th century. 6. Women in medicine – Great Britain – History – 16th century. 7. Women in medicine – Great Britain – History – 17th century. 8. Botany, Medical – Great Britain – History – 16th century. 9. Botany, Medical – Great Britain – History – 17th century. I. Title.
PR113.L36 2010
820'.9'9287–dc22 2009020468

ISBN 978-0-7546-6678-3

Mixed Sources
Product group from well-managed forests and other controlled sources
www.fsc.org Cert no. SA-COC-1565
© 1996 Forest Stewardship Council
FSC

Printed and bound in Great Britain by
MPG Books Group, UK

For my mother, Ruth Lambert,
who knows where the wild ginger grows,
and my father, Andre Laroche,
who can name every tree.

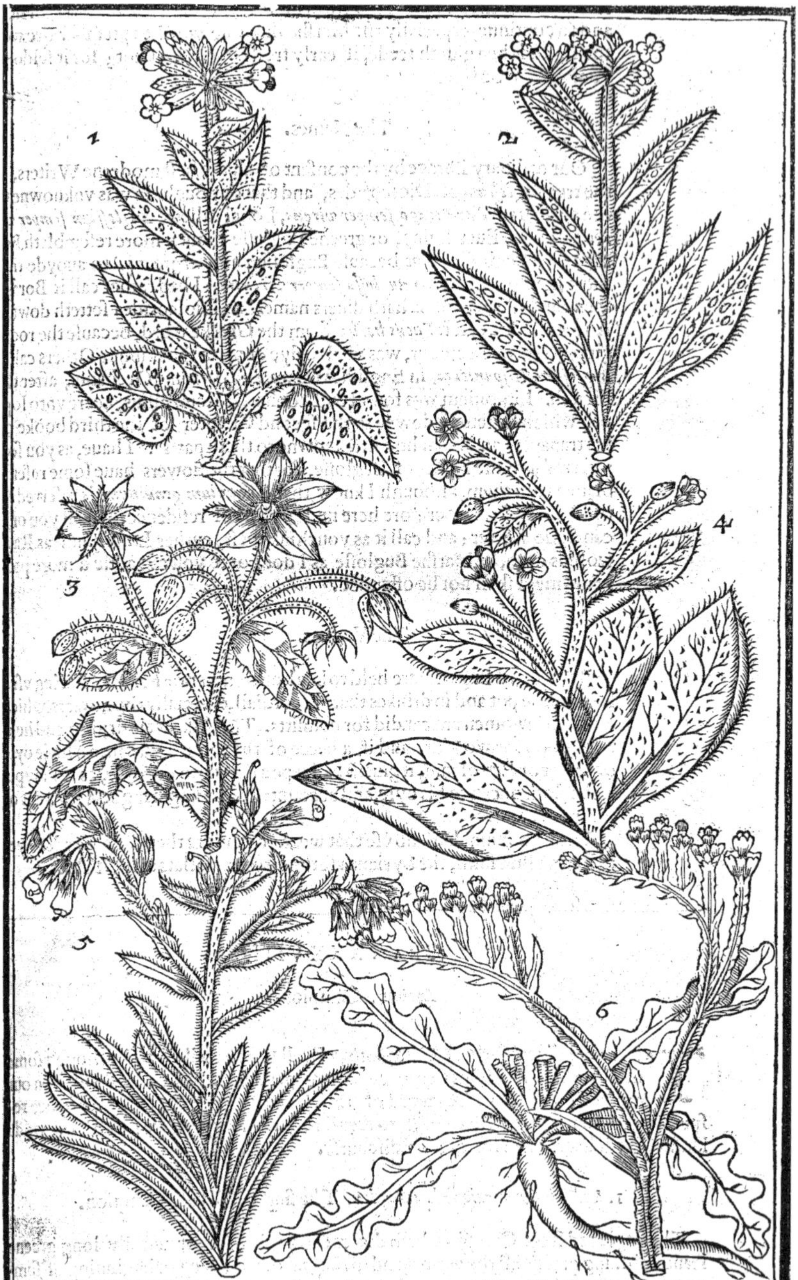

Image of Borage from John Parkinson's *Paradisi in Sole Paradisus Terrestris* (1629). By permission of the Cushing Rare Book and Manuscript Library.

Contents

List of Figures

Acknowledgments

To the following individuals and scholarly organizations I am very grateful, for they have maintained my intellectual health in the past seven years of research and writing and without their wholesome influence this book would have weakened, worsened, and wasted away: I start with my home department at the University of Colorado at Colorado Springs, especially Susan Taylor, who was English Department chair during my research time. These colleagues accommodated my research leaves and articulated support in many other ways. In sponsoring one of my leaves, The Institute for the Medical Humanities at the University of Texas Medical Branch and its generous climate of dialogue were invaluable in the spring and summer of 2007. I think of the Institute often and wish it and Galveston in general a sustained recovery from Hurricane Ike. Another major influence has been friend and mentor Bill Sheidley who, in reading the entire manuscript and expressing his excitement about the outcome, has kept me going through sometimes stressful final revisions.

Other residential fellowships and granting bodies have provided essential support in crucial stages from beginning to end, and I thank those who helped me gain this support by writing letters and reading prosposals. When the idea was just a seed needing roots, the Committee for Research and Creative Work and the Women's Faculty Committee at UCCS both provided monies for me to spend some time in the archive. Newly sprouted, the project received fertilization from the Huntington, Folger Shakespeare, and Beinecke Libraries through residencies at those venerable institutions, where fruitful conversations with other scholars often opened up new ways of thinking. The librarians at these and dozens of other libraries across the country and in Britain, whom I have tried to acknowledge throughout the individual chapters, have been essential. Finally, two other groups brought my research into full flowering through the exchange of ideas. Summer 2005, I participated in the National Endowment for the Humanities Summer Institute at the Folger, "The Handwritten Worlds of Early Modern England," and found myself in a community of thinkers that continues to inspire me. Then in September 2007, I participated in the workshop "Constructing Elizabeth Isham," without which the book would lack a most crucial figure. I thank Steven May and Kathleen Lynch, and Erica Longfellow and Elizabeth Clarke, respectively, for including me.

Those who have helped in giving the research, I hope, some perennial power are Rebecca Bushnell, Minette Church, Alix Cooper, Julie Eckerle, Raphael Falco, Jason Glenn, Christina Jimenez, William Kerwin, Mary Ellen Lamb, Lawrence Manley, Steven Mentz, Jennifer Munroe, Kate Narveson, Patricia Parker, Gail Kern Paster, Fred Schurink and Kimbra Smith, who all read prospectuses for the project and critiqued chapters that actually made it into the book, and I am grateful to those who read pieces that did not (though I hope I will have other occasions to thank them). Special thanks to Shannon Miller for her work as my research assistant. In general, I have been very lucky in my students, who in participating in senior seminars on the topics of early modern women, medicine, and literature, have renewed my energy repeatedly and shown me once again the symbiotic nature of the several parts of my occupation. And I have been luckier still in Ashgate's Erika Gaffney, whose patience and work ethic rival anyone's in her position.

Finally, previous versions of some of the material included in this study have appeared in *New Ways of Looking at Old Texts IV*, *Notes and Queries*, *The Yale University Library Gazette*, *A Manuscript Miscellany* (a Folger Institute website), and the *Constructing Elizabeth Isham* site, and I appreciate the work of those fora in initially publishing my scholarship and in giving me the rights to reprint it here.

Introduction
Medical Authority and Englishwomen's Herbal Texts, 1550–1650

The Herball or Generall Historie of Plantes by John Gerard, first published in 1597, lists more than twenty-six medicinal uses for rue, or the "herbe Grace." Purportedly the plant "prouoketh vrine," remedies testicle hardening, alleviates stomach "windines," helps joint pain, reduces spleen swelling, "killeth the shingles," eases an earache, sharpens eyesight, and stops a nosebleed. It can be used "with good successe against the dropsie," ague fits, and poisonings, and is seen as a cough medicine and an abortifacient as well as a preventative against the plague. In order to attain these benefits, the reader of Gerard's *Herball* must execute a number of processes after buying or harvesting this herb. It may be boiled with vinegar or with other plants (e.g., bay leaves, fenugreek, or dill), made into a poultice or ointment by adding it to grease or fat, combined with and preserved in oil, formed into a suppository, mixed with honey or wine, pressed for its juice, heated "in the rinde of a Pomegranate," ground into a paste with figs, administered in a clyster, warmed in the sun, ground, beaten, scalded, or pickled.[1] In addition to choosing a treatment, the practitioner must be able to discern different kinds of rue, as some wild varieties have poisonous potentials.

Even though early modernity referred to such practice as "simpling," it is clear from this example that there is nothing simple about it. That two different readers may approach this treatise on plants and their medicinal uses for different purposes and with different skill sets is also clear. That there is such variety and complexity is one of the reasons for the herbal's existence in the first place. No matter how extensive one's hands-on experience with medical plants, the herbal offered knowledge beyond individual and local experience. Thus it was highly prized not only for the material cost of its much-illustrated folio production but also for its usefulness.[2]

It is the usefulness of the herbal that interests us here; that is, in this study, we will read our herbals with a difference. We will not turn to the early modern herbal for added meaning to occasional Shakespearean references but actually ask about the significance of the books themselves. The herbal will not be viewed

---

[1] John Gerard, *The Herball or Generall Historie of Plantes* (London, 1597), 1070–76. Subsequent citations included in the text.

[2] See William Sherman's discussion of the Marxist distinction between "use value" and "exchange value" as it applies to the treatment of books, *Used Books: Marking Readers in Renaissance England* (Philadelphia: University of Pennsylvania Press, 2008), 177–78.

simply as a reference text to buttress our twenty-first-century understanding that Ophelia, in her gesture to Gertrude, points to their sexualized bodies in rue's abortifacient qualities or that Helena, dubbed the "herb of grace" by Lavatch, is the panacea of the play's ills.[3] Rather, our herbals are functional texts frequently found in the early modern household. That these resources were often owned and used by women is the prime mover of my analysis, and I hope this focus will advance our understanding of early modern Englishwomen's engagement with herbal signifiers and thus medical authority. I hope it will do so, however, not by making generalizations about early modern women's uses of these texts, but rather in uncovering and analyzing the various kinds of evidence and multiple contexts for these uses.

Women and Medical Authority

My belief in the fruitfulness of the general ground of early modern women's herbalism in part grows out of the inspirational research undertaken by historians in the past century that seeks to delineate women's medicine within the field of medical history. The statistical, archival, anthropological, and sociological work undertaken by Lucinda McCray Beier, Elizabeth Lane Furdell, Elaine Hobby, Lynette Hunter, Kate Campbell Hurd-Mead, Doreen Evenden Nagy, Margaret Pelling, Sara Pennell, Roy Porter, Rebecca Tannenbaum, Andrew Wear, and Charles Webster, to name a dozen, have identified over one hundred separate women undertaking some form of practice—whether as midwives, gentlewomen practitioners, housewives, herbwomen, wisewomen, witches, or empirics—in the sixteenth and seventeenth centuries.[4] The evidence they have cited comes from

[3] Current discussions of Ophelia's herbs point to the "antifertility" aspects of many of the herbs she carries; see Robert Painter and Brian Parker, "Ophelia's Flowers Again," *Notes and Queries* 239.1 (March 1994): 42–43. Lavatch's equation of Helena with "sweet marjoram" and then the "herb of grace" in Act IV scene 5 points to her position as healing but not healer; *All's Well That Ends Well*, in *The Norton Shakespeare*, ed. Stephen Greenblatt et al. (New York: W. W. Norton, 1997), 4.5.14–15.

[4] Lucinda McCray Beier, *Sufferers and Healers: The Experience of Illness in Seventeenth-Century England* (London: Routledge & Kegan Paul, 1987); Elizabeth Lane Furdell, *Publishing and Medicine in Early Modern England* (Rochester, New York: University of Rochester Press, 2002); Elaine Hobby, *Virtue of Necessity: English Women's Writing, 1649–88* (Ann Arbor: University of Michigan Press, 1989); Lynette Hunter, "Women and Domestic Medicine: Lady Experimenters, 1570–1620," in *Women, Science and Medicine 1500–1700: Mothers and Sisters of the Royal Society*, ed. Lynette Hunter and Sarah Hutton (Stroud, Gloucestershire: Sutton Publishing, 1997), 89–107; Kate Campbell Hurd-Mead, *A History of Women in Medicine, from the Earliest Times to the Beginning of the Nineteenth Century* (Haddam, Connecticut: The Haddam Press, 1938); Doreen Evenden Nagy, *Popular Medicine in Seventeenth-Century England* (Bowling Green, Ohio: Bowling Green State University Popular Press, 1988); Margaret Pelling (with Frances White), *Medical*

diaries, memoirs, manuscript and print recipe books, print manuals, inscriptions, memorials, wills, and historical records. Even though much of this evidence points to the charitable contributions of gentlewomen to the health of the poor, the women these historians name come from all stations. Then again, each historian admits that those of lesser economic status are more difficult to identify—the annals of the College of Physicians most regularly testifying (and most always in a negative light) to their presence. Research, however, continues to uncover new resources for such inquiry into women's history and, in the end, this study attempts to consider the difference economic status can make.

In tandem with an alternative articulation of the "medical marketplace," the findings of these historians intercede in a discussion of medical practice dependent upon a "tripartite division" of medical authority, which puts the physician at the top, with surgeons and apothecaries usually figuring underneath. Any overinvestment in such an establishment, whatever the motivations, is thus rightly challenged.[5] Margaret Pelling writes that

> selected institutions of the early modern period and before have been made to carry a considerable burden of interpretation. The reality of the tripartite division of medicine in England depends on the universal significance of certain well-known developments in the institutionalisation of medicine in London: the foundation of the College of Physicians . . . in 1518; the merging of the Barbers' Company with the tiny elite of the surgeons in 1540; and the splitting off of the Apothecaries from the Grocers Company in 1617.[6]

Conflicts in Early Modern London: Patronage, Physicians, and Irregular Practitioners, 1550–1640 (Oxford: Clarendon Press, 2003); Elaine Leong and Sara Pennell, "Recipe Collections and the Currency of Medical Knowledge in the Early Modern 'Medical Marketplace,'" in *Medicine and the Market in England and Its Colonies, c. 1450–c.1850*, ed. Mark S. R. Jenner and Patrick Wallis (Basingstoke, Hampshire: Palgrave Macmillan, 2007), 133–52; Roy Porter, *Health for Sale: Quackery in England 1660–1850* (Manchester: Manchester University Press, 1989); Rebecca Tannenbaum, *The Healer's Calling: Women and Medicine in Early New England* (Ithaca, New York: Cornell University Press, 2002); Andrew Wear, *Knowledge and Practice in English Medicine, 1550–1680* (Cambridge: Cambridge University Press, 2000); and Margaret Pelling and Charles Webster, "Medical Practitioners," *Health, Medicine and Mortality in the Sixteenth Century* (Cambridge: Cambridge University Press, 1979), 165–236. See also Monica H. Green, *Making Women's Medicine Masculine: The Rise of Male Authority in Pre-Modern Gynaecology* (Oxford: Oxford University Press, 2008), and cases cited by Deborah E. Harkness in *The Jewel House: Elizabethan London and the Scientific Revolution* (New Haven, Connecticut: Yale University Press, 2007), 63–75.

5 For an account of the emergence of the "medical marketplace" in discussions of medical history, see Mark S. R. Jenner and Patrick Wallis, eds., "The Medical Marketplace," in *Medicine and the Market*, 1–22.

6 Margaret Pelling, "Trade or Profession? Medical Practice in Early Modern England," in *The Common Lot: Sickness, Medical Occupations and the Urban Poor in Early Modern*

The main effect of an investment in the physician–surgeon–apothecary set of practitioners, which seldom, if ever, allowed for female participants, is the idea that—with rare exception—medicine belonged in the hands of men. The work of the historians mentioned above has proven that this is not the case. My analysis, in line with Pelling's, asks us to further lift the burden from this three-part structure and thus uncover potentials beyond inside and outside, legitimate and illegitimate, and open the medical model so that it better reflects the participation of women.

It is important to interrogate literary and cultural criticism's previous investment in the three-part system. Of course, the model in question is quite masculinist and elitist, one that, in focusing on health care provided by educated and licensed men centered in London, excludes the contributions of female, unaffiliated, and rural contributors. An investment in such a model may come from what Pelling calls a "positivist" stance, in which the early modern moment is seen as the beginning of the advances found in modern organized medicine, with the most important early modern components persisting today.[7] This positivism would explain why, before William Kerwin's recent reading of Helena in *All's Well That Ends Well* in the context of women practitioners brought before the College of Physicians, scholarly discussions of medicine in *All's Well* focused on the Galenic versus Paracelsian debate among early modern male physicians.[8]

From a different vantage, the tripartite division provides a system of repressive hierarchies that supports a narrative of the subjugation of women, a key component of the system being its exclusion of female practitioners; therefore, in early feminist assessments of medicine in early modern England such as those by Jeanne Achterberg, Barbara Ehrenreich, and Deirdre English, the physician–apothecary–surgeon triad supplies the authorized and authorizing inside to which the female and poor constituted the persecuted and stigmatized outside.[9] As we will find out

---

England (Harlow, Essex: Longman, 1998), 235.

7 Pelling, "Trade or Profession?" 230.

8 William Kerwin, "Medea's Traces: Women Practitioners in History and Drama," in *Beyond the Body: The Boundaries of Medicine and English Renaissance Drama* (Amherst: University of Massachusetts Press, 2005), 62–96. Richard K. Stensgaard, "All's Well That Ends Well and the Galenico-Paracelsian Controversy," *Renaissance Quarterly* 25.2 (Summer 1972), 173–88, and Henry D. Janowitz,"Helena's Medicine in *All's Well that Ends Well*: Is it Paracelsian or Hermetical in Origin?" *Cauda Pavonis: Studies in Hermeticism* 20.1 (2001 Spring), 20–22. Since Kerwin's publication, Catherine Field's essay, "'Sweet Practicer, thy Physic I will try': Helena and her 'Good Receipt' in *All's Well, That Ends Well*," in *All's Well, That Ends Well: New Critical Essays*, ed. Gary Waller (New York: Routledge, 2007), 194–208, has also contributed to our understanding of Helena by adding the context of women's recipe books. See also Todd H. J. Pettigrew, *Shakespeare and the Practice of Physic: Medical Narratives on the Early Modern English Stage* (Newark: University of Delaware Press, 2007).

9 Jeanne Achterberg, *Woman as Healer* (Boston: Shambhala Press, 1991), 78–85; Barbara Ehrenreich and Deirdre English, *Witches, Midwives, and Nurses: A History of Women Healers* (Old Westbury, New York: The Feminist Press, 1973), 17–19. For a

in our discussion of Isabella Whitney, this is not a narrative that exists solely in second-wave feminist accounts, but it is one that applies in specific contexts and to particular ends. My project here follows the work of Margaret Ezell, Phyllis Rackin, and others, who have asked us to reevaluate some of the assumptions embedded in earlier feminist interpretive models, in particular those that focus on the subjugation of women.[10]

Ironically, the narrative of exclusion and subjugation solidifies a tripartite division that was not historically in place. Pelling tells us, "Taken as a whole, medical practice in early modern England was neither well organized nor firmly controlled. No system of surveillance had more than partial application. The tripartite structure more strictly adopted in continental Europe remained the aim of minority groups,"[11] and historians after her have consequently shown a medical market that is much more fluid and responsive to patient demands.[12] One important means of stepping away from this structure would be to look squarely at the "minority groups" in early modern England who were invested in this system, and throughout this study, we turn to moments that reflect the desire for the goal of "firm control" in order to assess the reasons for the investment in control at that particular moment. Many such occasions can be found in the establishment of the authoritative print herbal tradition, an establishment which we will study at length in this project's first chapter.

Like corresponding literary traditions, the herbal had an extensive life in print on the Continent before coming to England. In Germany, Italy, and the Spanish Lowlands, influential treatises had been published by Leonhart Fuchs, Pietro Mattioli, Rembert Dodoens, and many others. This print life grew out of extensive manuscript preservation of classical texts, most commonly those by Dioscorides and Pliny, before them. In England, the key figures known for establishing the authoritative vernacular herbal tradition, particularly as they come to be invoked in the later volumes, were William Turner, Henry Lyte (as translator of Dodoens), John Gerard, and John Parkinson. Their dates of publication roughly frame this study. While these folios had their place in the history of botany, they also had a practical application in enabling lay medical practice by both men and women.

The sometimes reluctant acknowledgment in these volumes of women's practice in herbalism provides a fascinating point of analysis for the establishment of the authoritative tradition. In Chapter 1, we discover that the English vernacular herbal tradition, similar to its literary analogues, struggles with a belated entrée

---

critique of such myth-making see Diane Purkiss, *The Witch in History: Early Modern and Twentieth-Century Representations* (Routledge: London, 1996).

10 Margaret J. M. Ezell, *Writing Women's Literary History* (Baltimore: Johns Hopkins University Press, 1993); Phyllis Rackin, *Shakespeare and Women* (Oxford: Oxford University Press, 2005).

11 Pelling, "Trade or Profession?" 244.

12 See Harkness, *The Jewel House*, and Jenner and Wallis, eds., *Medicine and the Market*.

relative to its continental counterparts and, as it becomes established, articulates anxieties about individual competitors within the English tradition. Given current understandings of Western literary traditions, it should not be surprising that it voices these anxieties through gendered language. An example of one looking to establish the tight "control" of a "tripartite" system, William Turner, a physician now commonly known as the "Father of English Botany,"[13] writes to exclude the herbwives—gatherers and sellers of herbs—from the circulation of herbal knowledge, publishing his herbal so that others, like himself, would be "not trustinge onlye to the olde herbe wiues" (sig.*3r). However, as we will discuss at greater length in the next chapter, when Turner writes this passage, it comes at a moment in the framing of his herbal project that communicates unease about his belated position with relation to his continental precursors (who have a better-established "system of surveillance") and the fallibility of the textual tradition.[14] The full analysis follows to some extent the work of Steven Shapin (and after him Rebecca Bushnell), who shows how male authors establish roles as "truth-tellers" in part through the scapegoating of "old wives,"[15] but with this project's second and third chapters, which focus on women who actually owned the authoritative text, my analysis goes on to demonstrate how this establishment of truth is destabilized by the presence of the woman reader. In the circulation of knowledge through the printed text, women became owners of the textual truth that was then modified and recontextualized in their experience. One can imagine that those invested in institutional regulation were those who would be the controllers, not those who would be controlled; moreover, my research here, along with that of the historians listed above, demonstrates how, across a population, even though there were individuals who were subject to regulation and censure, there were other women for whom such strictures never applied. Thus it is important to consider the moments that invoke regulation—and these can be either male- or female-authored—as particular to the text at hand rather than indicative of an overall oppressive model. In doing so, we uncover the specific ways that women engaged herbal texts in order to invoke or confound medical authority, and we find that medical authority as represented was either established or in flux within any given context: that is, medical practice was either highly hierarchized and regulated or freely practiced and highly diversified, depending on the context of its representation. While this contingency is certainly hinted at by the work of the above historians, literary critics have yet to explore fully its implications.

The richness of the findings about historical women's practice has indeed moved literary critics to call upon the names of Nagy and Pelling in their analysis

---

[13] For an account of the title in twentieth-century analysis, see Chapter 1, n. 5.

[14] William Turner, *The Seconde Parte of VVilliam Turners Herball* (Cologne, 1562).

[15] Steven Shapin, *A Social History of Truth: Civility and Science in Seventeenth-Century England* (Chicago: The University of Chicago Press, 1994), 90; Rebecca Bushnell, *Green Desire: Imagining Early Modern English Gardens* (Ithaca, New York: Cornell University Press, 2003), 177.

of literature. Before now, however, any book-length study has focused on early modern drama; thus, because of relatively few extant dramas by women, we have yet to consider closely female-authored texts. Recent monograph studies by William Kerwin and Wendy Wall and the collection *Disease, Diagnosis, and Cure on the Early Modern Stage*, edited by Stephanie Moss and Kaara Peterson, make good use of these historical findings while adding to our understanding of the dramatic materials.[16] The broader concern in each of these books on domesticity or general medicine relegates the issue of women's medical practice to discrete chapters and presents women's herbalism only as evidence of the more general domestic practice. My goal is to further develop insights gained in these differently focused chapters within the specific contexts of herbalism and women's writing.

Alternatively, within the subfield of early modern women writers, analyses of female-authored texts such as Whitney's *Sweet Nosgay* (1573) (the subject of Chapter 4) and Anne Wheathill's *A handfull of holesome (though homelie) hearbs* (1584) that invoke historical research have only yet done so in glosses or digressions, and, as a result, they tend to generalize about women's medical practice without considering the differences that the individual text may reflect.[17] In the main, the

[16] Kerwin, *Beyond the Body*; Wendy Wall, *Staging Domesticity: Household Work and English Identity in Early Modern Drama* (Cambridge: Cambridge University Press, 2002); Stephanie Moss and Kaara L. Peterson, eds., *Disease, Diagnosis, and Cure on the Early Modern Stage* (Burlington, Vermont: Ashgate Publishing, 2004). See also Pettigrew, *Shakespeare and the Practice of Physic*, and Tanya Pollard, *Drugs and Theater in Early Modern England* (Oxford: Oxford University Press, 2005).

A female-authored dramatic episode that speaks to women's practice can be found in Elizabeth Cavendish Brackley's and Jane Cavendish's *The Concealed Fancies*, Act III, scene 4, in which three female cousins enter their uncle's closet and discover his herbal distillations and "a whole box of my Lady Kent's cordials," in *Renaissance Drama by Women: Texts and Documents*, ed. S. P. Cerasano and Marion Wynne-Davies (London: Routledge, 1996), 3.4.56–57. My thanks to Christina Luckyj for drawing my attention to this episode.

[17] For examples, see Colin B. Atkinson and Jo B. Atkinson, "Anne Wheathill's *A Handfull of Holesome (though Homelie) Hearbs* (1584): The First English Gentlewoman's Prayer Book," *The Sixteenth Century Journal* 27.3 (Fall 1996): 659–72; Wendy Wall, "Authorship and the Material Conditions of Writing," in *The Cambridge Companion to English Literature, 1500–1600*, ed. Arthur F. Kinney (Cambridge: Cambridge University Press, 2000), 64–89; and Jennifer Wynne Hellwarth, "'Be unto me as a precious ointment: Lady Grace Mildmay, Sixteenth-Century Female Practitioner," *Dynamis* 19 (1999): 95–117. An exception that explores the trope a bit more at length is Susan Felch's analysis of Ann Vaughan Lock's "authorial medicine" in the 1560 printing of her translations of Calvin, "Ann Lock's Authorial Medicine," *Reformation* 2 (1997): 7–38. Another exception is Richelle Munkoff's treatment of Rachel Speght's medicinal content in light of her findings about female searchers in early modern London (seminar paper contributed at the meeting of the Shakespeare Association of America, Victoria, British Columbia, April 10–12, 2003), which points to diversity in women's practice but is part of a project that is not on women's medicine in general; Richelle Munkhoff, "Searchers of the Dead: Authority, Marginality,

effect of historical findings regarding women's practice on the study of female-authored texts has been the limitation of those texts. That is, much of the evidence presented by the above historians has come in the form of texts written by women, and as a result, in a particularly circular fashion, any mention of medicine in those texts is explained—and later invoked—as simply historical fact. Indicative of this practice is the regularity with which two women, Lady Margaret Hoby and Lady Grace Mildmay, are named in the lists of historical examples establishing women's practice (one or both are named in almost all of the historical and literary studies cited so far). Hoby's diary and Mildmay's written remains—which include a brief autobiography, devotional meditations, and hundreds of pages of medical recipes—provide ample illustrations of women's medical education and practice, and both have a prominent place in this study's third chapter, but in that chapter, the herbal content in both diary and autobiography will not be considered only as historical evidence. Rather, when we consider these works critically, the represented episode of reading the herbal tells us as much about the text it is a part of as it does about the woman's practice. As a result, these writings are not examined here as they are typically alongside other later examples of Anne Halkett and Lucy Hutchinson, who also give evidence in their autobiographical writings of women's practice but not of women's herbal reading.[18] What is more, when examining these texts next to each other (and both of them next to the more recently discovered example of Elizabeth Isham), it becomes very clear that they tell us quite different things about access to medical care and the gendering of herbal authority. In returning to textual moments previously regarded mainly as historical evidence, we may find added meaning within the historical "realities" of women's herbalisms.

Indicative of the instability of these realities is the presence of the print herbal itself. Even though some of the herbalists may have asserted an authoritative control over their readership, there is no way to insure that any control actually existed. In creating a kind of portable authority for an English-literate audience, these volumes provided a means for the owner to become an herbal authority. Moreover, anticipating late seventeenth-century works studied by Adrian Johns and as discussed below and in Chapter 4, a number of "epitomes" derived from these larger volumes existing both in print and manuscript dislocated the authority from the source, further authorizing the work of the reader.[19] Thus, for the practitioner, the knowledge of herbs and their medical benefits was available through networks

and the Interpretation of Plague in England, 1574–1665," *Gender & History* 11.1 (April 1999): 1–29. I have presented on Wheathill's herbalism in several fora, but as I see her engagement as mainly with devotional texts rather than medical ones, I have separated a discussion of her work from this monograph study.

[18] Anne Halkett, *The Memoirs of Anne, Lady Halkett and Ann, Lady Fanshawe*, ed. John Loftis (Oxford: Clarendon Press, 1979); and Lucy Hutchinson, *Memoirs of the Life of Colonel Hutchinson*, ed. James Sutherland (London: Oxford University Press, 1973).

[19] Adrian Johns, *The Nature of the Book: Print and Knowledge in the Making* (Chicago: University of Chicago Press, 1998).

of derivative texts and other practitioners. By presenting together herbal treatises and female-authored texts as objects for analysis, this study demonstrates how both male-authored and female-authored writings represent women's herbal practice as constituting various relationships with medical authority, which itself was paradoxically both solidified and made fluid through publication.

It is in exploring women's engagement with print herbals that this study looks to recent advancements in the History of the Book and the History of Reading, particularly those studies that consider the female "reader's place within the literary transaction."[20] Heidi Brayman Hackel, Kathryn DeZur, Mary Erler, Mary Ellen Lamb, Paul Morgan, Sasha Roberts, William Sherman, and Edith Snook all articulate and analyze the position of the woman reader.[21] In doing so, they have given texture to debates about female literacy, advanced our conception of a gendered intellect, and highlighted names that were otherwise obscured in the archives. *Englishwomen's Herbal Texts* looks to contribute to this endeavor by shedding light on the particular instances in which women read texts that provided herbal remedy and in the process articulated some relationship to medical authority. Thus here the "literary transaction" is framed in specifically medicinal terms.

While this is not a study of Englishwomen writers that sets out to make generalizations about women's experience and their representations thereof, it does center on women's texts and does so for several reasons. Most importantly, if

---

20 Kathryn DeZur, "'Vaine Books' and Early Modern Women Readers," in *Reading and Literacy in the Middle Ages and Renaissance*, ed. Ian Frederick Moulton (Turnhout, Belgium: Brepols, 2004), 105.

21 Heidi Brayman Hackel, *Reading Material in Early Modern England: Print, Gender, and Literacy* (Cambridge: Cambridge University Press, 2005); DeZur, "'Vaine Books'"; Mary C. Erler, *Women, Reading, and Piety in Late Medieval England* (Cambridge: Cambridge University Press, 2002); Mary Ellen Lamb, "Constructions of Women Readers," in *Teaching Tudor and Stuart Women Writers*, ed. Susanne Woods and Margaret P. Hannay (New York: Modern Language Association of America; 2000), 23–34, and (more specifically) "Margaret Hoby's Diary: Women's Reading Practices and the Gendering of the Reformation Subject," *Pilgrimage for Love: Essays in Early Modern Literature in Honor of Josephine A. Roberts*, ed. Sigrid King (Tempe, Arizona: Center for Medieval and Renaissance Studies, 1999), 63–94; Paul Morgan, "Frances Wolfreston and 'Hor Bouks': A Seventeenth-Century Woman Book-Collector," *The Library* 6.2 (1989): 197–219; Sasha Roberts, *Reading Shakespeare's Poems in Early Modern England* (Basingstoke, Hampshire: Palgrave Macmillan, 2003); William Sherman, "Reading the Matriarchive," in *Used Books*, 53–67; and Edith Snook, *Women, Reading, and the Cultural Politics of Early Modern England* (Aldersho, Hampshiret: Ashgate Publishing, 2005). See also Ezell, *Writing Women's Literary History*, and Stephen Orgel, "Marginal Maternity: Reading Lady Anne Clifford's *A Mirror for Magistrates*," in *Printing and Parenting in Early Modern England*, ed. Douglas A. Brooks (Burlington, Vermont: Ashgate Publishing, 2005), 267–89. The collection edited by Heidi Brayman Hackel and Catherine E. Kelly, *Reading Women: Literacy, Authorship and Culture in the Atlantic World, 1500–1800* (Philadelphia: University of Pennsylvania Press, 2008), furthers this conversation as well.

female-authored texts are to gain equal footing in the discussion of early modern English culture, the terms of inquiry must change. Whereas discussions of literary traditions as established by nineteenth-century scholars continue to keep sixteenth- and seventeenth-century female writers in belated or marginal positions,[22] I believe that analysis with an eye toward herbal content may uncover interesting potentials in works by writers of either gender. I have chosen to concentrate on the range of textual possibilities relative to women's herbal practice and their engagement with herbal texts, which was as consistent as—if less established than—men's practice, because I do not want this to be a discussion of differences between genders (which would incline toward essentialism) but one that rather considers variables such as economic and marital status and geographical location that exist alongside gender.[23] Neither women's writing nor their medical practice is thus seen to be monolithic.

In essence, my analysis looks to elucidate the variety of cultural implications occurring when women engage with herbal texts and thereby claim some relationship to medical practice. After examining the print herbal tradition itself and establishing the social networks at play in women's ownership as indicated through their inscriptions in the books, I consider four instances of female authors (Margaret Hoby, Grace Mildmay, Elizabeth Isham, and Isabella Whitney) who reference various herbal texts in their writings. In thus appropriating herbal texts, each woman represents more and other than the general cultural phenomenon of women's medicine. In considering women of varying social position, marital status, and geographic origin, and works in both manuscript and print, this study draws on the "cultural historical approach" of Roger Chartier, one that "focuses on differentiated practices and contrasted uses" and thus "accentuates plural uses and diverse readings which are not aimed at or inscribed in the text."[24] This approach allows us to see that there are many factors affecting women's engagement with herbalism, not the least of which is the kind of text (authoritative or affordable) she may choose to consult in the pursuit of knowledge. These variable practices and uses thus provide a constellation of women's histories surrounding a single theme.

---

22 Ezell, *Writing Women's Literary History*. See also Rebecca Laroche, "Pamphilia Across a Crowded Room: Mary Wroth's Entry into the Canon," *Genre* 30.4 (Winter 1997), 267–88.

23 Karen Reeds is currently working on a survey of different early modern uses of the herbal as evidenced in inscriptions and marginalia, and is presenting this work in different venues. For example, she has recently delivered a paper at the colloquium "Theory and Practice in Ancient and Medieval Medicine: A Seminar in Honor of John Riddle" at the Institute of Medieval Studies, University of New Mexico, Albuquerque, Oct. 24/25, 2008. For her work leading up to this current path of study, see *Botany in Medieval and Renaissance Universities* (New York: Garland Publishing, 1991).

24 Roger Chartier, *Cultural History: Between Practices and Representations,* trans. Lydia G. Cochrane (Ithaca, New York: Cornell University Press, 1988), 13.

It is in the interest of representing such differentiation that I will conclude this introductory chapter with a discussion of three separate instances of women reading Gerard's *Herball*. These three instances differ in the frame in which Gerard's text appears and the ways in which the female reader asserts or erases the herbal author's and/or her own presence. Each of the examples raises the question of audience, either as an audience is defined by Gerard or as it is reconstructed by the woman reading Gerard. As a result, these examples begin our discussion of the variety of economic, sociological, and textual factors that inform women's engagement with an authoritative herbal, and in light of these factors, the herbal comes to take on various and unexpected significances.

Selections from Gerard and the Question of Audience

As an object in and of itself, Gerard's *Herball*, in its authoritative and literal weight, may be seen to represent metonymically a kind of medical authority reflective of the "tripartite division" discussed earlier. Gerard himself was a surgeon, and his position as the gardener of William Cecil, Lord Burghley, certainly gave his text a kind of official stamp. We can see this authoritativeness throughout the volume, particularly in its paratextual elements written to and by physicians, courtiers, and other men of note as well as in the moments in which the author breaks from the mode of mere transmission of information and directly addresses his reader. We may interrogate this medical authority as it is thus textually represented through the first woman's text to be discussed here, which not coincidentally interacts with one of those moments when the author steps outside the frame.

The following recipe "To make Gerrards excellent Balsome" can be found in a manuscript entitled "RECEIPTS APPROVED BY PERSONS of qualitie and iudgment, collected by Elizabeth Digby: 1650":

> Take oyle of Roses, oyle of St Johns-worte, of each a pinte; of the leaves of tobacco stamped small in a stone morter two pounds: boyle them together to the consumption of the iuice; straine it, and put it to the fire againe, adding thereto of Venus Turpen=tine two ounces; Olbaine [Olibanum] and Masticke, of each ~~f~~halfe an ounce; in most fine and subtill powder: Herewith you may at all times make an unguent or Salve by putting thereto waxe and Rosin, to give it a stiffe body; which worketh exceeding well in malignat [*sic*] and virulent ~~humours~~ ulcers, as in wounds & punctions. This Balsome is excellent to cure deepe wounds and puncti=one made by some narrow sharpe pointed weapon; which Balsome doth up the flesh from the bottome very speedily; and also healeth small cutts in flesh: It doth conglutinate the lippes of wounds together, not procuring matter or corruption unto it, as is com[m]only seene in healing of wounds.[25]

[25] Elizabeth Digby, "Receipts of Elizabeth Digby," British Library MS Egerton 2197, 23r, in *Defining Gender, 1450–1910* database, http://www.gender.amdigital.co.uk/contents/

Digby or another compiler before her has taken this recipe from Gerard's *Herball* (likely the 1597 version because it more closely reflects the punctuation from that edition) under the heading for tobacco or "Henbane of Peru" (286). Gerard's entry, in line with his list of the herb's "vertues" (the word used in the herbals to talk about a plant's medicinal benefits), begins with uses of the balsam. In the recipe collection, the author transposed the recipe with its use in order to align with other entries in her book, which all begin with the recipe itself and end with the disease that it helps alleviate. This transposition alone shows how the woman reader changed the text in reading it, transforming the herbal entry (listed as a virtue of tobacco) into a recipe (listed as how-to instructions). It is difficult to determine in this generic appropriation the extent to which the entry demonstrates Digby's direct engagement with Gerard; that is, if she has copied this from the recipe book of a compatriot, then the entry may not have so easily come to match her own format, but then again this format is shared by other examples in the recipe book genre. Regardless of whether Digby comes to Gerard's entry directly or copies it from someone else's copy, the recipe raises an intriguing array of possibilities surrounding one woman reader's engagement with medical authority as represented by the herbal author.

That is, although it is not immediately evident how this authority may be directly engaged, upon closer examination we find that the entry stops at an important juncture in Gerard's text, one before the author inserts his voice. After he gives this recipe, Gerard, in a rare moment in the herbal, turns directly to his female readership, which initially he describes as "women of all sorts" but then changes to "curteous gentlewomen":

> I send this iewell vnto you women of all sorts, especially to such as cure and helpe the poore and impotent of your countrie without rewarde. But vnto the beggerly rabble of witches, charmers, & such like couseners, that regarde more to get money then to helpe for charitie, I wish these fewe medicines far from their vnderstanding, and from those deceiuers whom I wish to bee ignoraunte heerein. But curteous gentlewomen, I may not for the malice that I doe beare vnto such, hide any thing from you of such importaunce. (288)

The original extended passage gives a context for the copying of the text: the writer of the recipe book entry may have been such a "curteous gentlewom[a]n" who practiced herbal remedy out of charity, and presumably Gerard's direct address drew the recipe to her attention. It also reveals to us how Gerard, as well as other herbal authors, conceived of his female readership. What it does not fully disclose is the purpose of including such a passage in a book that is not likely to be read by the "beggerly rabble" it derides, perhaps bringing to mind William Turner's herbwife, who, because of her illiteracy, is excluded from the circulation

image-viewing.aspx?imageid=44335 (accessed March 2, 2009). While staying true to original spelling, I have decided not to replicate or indicate line breaks.

of authorized herbal knowledge. In this way, Gerard forms his female reader by describing who she is not. Ironically, we may note that Digby's entry, in excluding this address to the female reader, leaves out Gerard's "wish" for the knowledge. In its manuscript circulation, this recipe holds none of the limitations or censures that its original print version upholds. So while the recipe retains the authority of Gerard through its title, its recontextualization within the recipe book of Elizabeth Digby allows for a wider variety of uses than to help "the poore and impotent." Whatever the reasoning for this omission (the most practical of course being the economy of paper), this one instance introduces the many possibilities of a reader's reception. A woman may read the herbal in cooperation with licensed medical authority (represented here by the "wish" of the surgeon John Gerard) or in the absence of such authority (represented here by the omission of his direct voice from the entry) or without a mind to that authority at all (in light of simple economy). Whatever the indeterminable authorial purposes may have been, the repositioning of the herbal passage within a particular woman's recipe book separates the passage from Gerard's aim and locates it more directly in line with Digby's uses.

Our second introductory example similarly takes in hand the problem of the presence or the absence of licensed authority within women's practice. Among the dozens of manuscript remedy books at the Wellcome Library in London—now conveniently available in microform—is one with a signature by a woman named Elizabeth Bulckley and with the title "A Booke of Hearbes & Receipts" and date 1627.[26] This volume—forty leaves, seven inches by five inches—is part of a subgenre within the remedy book category; unlike pure "receipt books" such as Digby's, collections of various cures of multiple ingredients from various oral, print, and manuscript sources, this remedy book starts out with a different inclination. Hand A, the same hand that writes the title and date but different from Bulckley's (Hand B), begins the book with more than twenty herbal entries that the writer distills from a larger print volume, again Gerard's 1597 *Herball or Generall Historie of Plantes*. As the volume seems largely constructed for and by women, I will refer to this writer, Compiler A, as "she" throughout my analysis. In this manuscript, Compiler A has copied out the "temperature," i.e., the Galenic qualities (hot or cold, moist or dry), of herbs such as mint, sage, thyme, and cowslip, and then each plant's "virtues" almost verbatim as they are described by Gerard, only condensed with abbreviations and some elisions; for example, "Wilde Time is of temperature hot and drie in the third degree" and "boiled in wine and drunke, is good against the wambling and gripings of the bellie" (457) becomes "Wilde tyme is hot & drye in the third degree," and "boyled in wine & drunke, is good against the wamblinge & gripings of the bellie" (fol. 5r). Notably,

---

[26] "A Booke of Hearbes & Receipts, 1627," Wellcome MS 169, in *Women and Medicine: Remedy Books, 1533–1865, from the Wellcome Library for the Understanding and History of Medicine*, ed. Sara Pennell (Reading: Primary Source Microfilm, Thomas Gale, 2004), Reel 1. Folio citations included in the text.

her concise and selected version of *The Herball* bears no overt reference to the male author in the manuscript. Gerard's name does not appear on the title page or within the herbal entries themselves. Only in incidental admonitions, such as an aside about "diuers rash & ouerboald Apothecaries, & other foolish weomen" (fol. 7r) is another authorial presence felt at all.

Because we currently know relatively little about Compiler A or the owner Elizabeth Bulckley, we can only imagine the criteria for the selection process, but we can infer from the indigenous and common quality of plants such as wild thyme and rosemary that it had something to do with the herbs that the first compiler had readily available. This hypothesis is in part supported when Compiler A has included entries for only red and white lilies out of the many varieties included in the herbal or has specified "Englishe Garlicke" when Gerard's entry is on garlic in general. This distillation of the herbal operates very differently from the later entries in the manuscript that appear as recipes (which are titled by the disease they cure, not the ingredient) and indicates the writer was someone pointedly interested in the cultivation and usage of herbs. The example of this handwritten condensed herbal also captures the act of reading; we can see how the recording of one herb, for example, garlic (Bulckley fol. 15v, Gerard 140–45), may have led to the record of the plant after it in Gerard's text, white garden lily (Bulckley fol. 16r, Gerard 146). Similarly, in the exclusion of the scholarly disputations, the growing conditions, and the discussion of the names of the plants and in their emphasis on the Galenic qualities and the plants' virtues, these herbal entries signify a medicinal use of herbs; the same hand that collected the entries implicitly also picked, processed, and applied each herb entered there.

Important feminist work has been undertaken in the past decade by a growing number of scholars including Robert Appelbaum, Michelle DiMeo, Catherine Field, Elaine Leong, Sara Pennell, and Jennifer Stine in the cataloging, reproduction, and analysis of manuscript receipt books, a genre invoked often in the establishment of women's medical practice.[27] As a result, we have learned

---

[27] Robert Appelbaum, "Rhetoric and Epistemology in Early Printed Recipe Collections," *Journal of Early Modern Cultural Studies* 3.2 (2003): 1–35; Michelle DiMeo, "The Draft of Elizabeth Isham's Medical Receipt Book," *Constructing Elizabeth Isham*, ed. Elizabeth Clarke and Erica Longfellow, http://www2.warwick.ac.uk/fac/arts/ren/projects/isham/workshop/dimeo/ (accessed June 13, 2008); and Catherine Field, "'Many hands hands': Writing the Self in Early Modern Women's Recipe Books," in *Genre and Women's Life Writing in Early Modern England*, ed. Michelle M. Dowd and Julie A. Eckerle (Burlington, Vermont: Ashgate Publishing, 2007), 49–64. Along with the introduction to the microfilm edition cited above, see Sara Pennell, "Perfecting Practice? Women, Manuscript Recipes, and Knowledge in Early Modern England," in *Early Modern Women's Manuscript Writing*, ed. Victoria E. Burke and Jonathan Gibson (Aldershot, Hampshire: Ashgate Publishing, 2004), 237–58, and Pennell's essay with Elaine Leong, "Recipe Collections and Medical Knowledge." See Leong's "Medical Recipe Collections in Seventeenth-Century England: Knowledge, Gender and Text" (Ph.D. diss., University of Oxford, 2005/06) and her introductory essay for *Receipt Books, c.1575–1800 from the Folger Shakespeare*

much about women's relationships to scientific experiment, architectural spaces, and learned communities. Indeed, plenty of work remains to be done. The *Perdita* database currently lists one hundred fourteen examples of women's recipe books, the majority of which include medical recipes, many of which have not yet been considered closely.[28] In some ways, a recipe book is the writing that is most directly related to medical practice, bearing witness to the practice in general and in the details, and, as Appelbaum has well explored, these collections have their own kind of rhetoric, one that is informed by the social practice they describe and the paratextual elements that frame them.[29] My focus intersects here with the discussion of recipe books through cases such as Digby's recipe and the Bulckley volume, when the remedy book entries bear some direct relation to the print herbal source, because, as we will see in more detail in Chapter 1, the print texts look to have a hand in the gendering of medical practice, and this gendering is then complicated by extensive reproduction of the text in a woman's hand as we find in the Bulckley remedy book.

In articulating the focus of the larger project, my particular interests in the Bulckley book are many. Yes, I am in part fascinated by the implicit medical practice behind the writing project, but I am also intrigued by the process of appropriation that Compiler A undertook in distilling Gerard's text. In this process, the knowledge published by Gerard now belonged to the woman compiling the remedy book. While some of the Englishwomen's texts examined here are authored by women who then gave their names to those texts, the second chapter of this study looks at the many instances in which women, by writing their names on titlepages or flyleaves, owned texts they did not author and through their ownership asserted a kind of "agency."[30] Moreover, in doing so, they often pointed to social contexts beyond the male-authored herbal. Bulckley's text also gives evidence of such agency and contexts.

What is more, unlike the late seventeenth-century example discussed at length by Elaine Leong and Raymond Anselment, Elizabeth Freke, who writes that each of her extensive manuscript sections is taken out of "Gerards" (often spelled "Geralds") herbal, and the above entry by Elizabeth Digby, "To make Gerrards excellent Balsome," the Bulckley Compiler A removes Gerard's name from the knowledge and, in the process of distillation or epitomization that occurs here,

---

Library, a microfilm publication (Marlborough, Wiltshire: Adam Matthew Publications, Ltd., 2006). See also Jennifer Stine, "Opening Closets: The Discovery of Household Medicine in Early Modern England" (Ph.D. diss., Stanford University, 1996).

28 *Perdita* database, dir. Elizabeth Clarke and Martyn Bennett, http://human.ntu.ac.uk/research/perdita/frames/html/index.htm (accessed March 9, 2009). See Leong and Pennell, "Recipe Collections and Medical Knowledge," for a general survey of the genre and an indication of more extensive work that has been done.

29 Appelbaum, "Rhetoric and Epistemology."

30 Orgel, "Marginal Maternity," 267.

dislocates knowledge from its authoritative source.[31] Adrian Johns has examined such epitomes in the realm of print, and many of those critics and historians working on recipe books and other manuscript miscellanies have considered the complex relationship between the print and handwritten volumes.[32] The relationship between manuscript herbal epitomes and their print sources is no less complex and is one that enacts a particular relationship to the medical authority involved. For example—and we will discuss this further below—the act of copying may be related to the process of learning; the repetition in writing helps to internalize the medical knowledge on the page. Also, in owning such knowledge, the writers to be examined articulate some association with medical authority, whether that authority is found only in print or in the practice of surgeons and physicians as well. Most importantly, and here I return to Chartier's conception of "differentiated practices," the practice of selection is also one of individuation. Leong and Pennell discuss "the processes of constructing personal medical knowledge" that occurs through recipe collections, and Field discusses the autobiographical elements in such compilations.[33] I would add that the "processes" of selection are not necessarily medical or self-reflexive but may also mirror the surrounding household and economic context. Not only does the knowledge now belong to the female practitioner, the herbs now belong specifically to her garden; another manuscript epitome of the same Gerard volume, another garden, would naturally include different herbs.[34] The Bulckley remedy book repositions the text within a new context, even though, admittedly, that context is only just discernible, since we lack not only a name for the compiler but also the biography of the named owner.

Thus "A Booke of Hearbes & Receipts" also introduces us to the frustrations and rewards of many of the instances examined in Chapter 2. Unlike the autobiographies of Hoby, Mildmay, and Isham considered in Chapter 3, many

---

[31] Elizabeth Freke, *The Remembrances of Elizabeth Freke, 1671–1714*, ed. Raymond A. Anselment (Cambridge: Cambridge University Press for the Royal Historical Society, 2001), 175, and Digby, "Receipts," 23r. While an important work to bring into dialogue with this study, such a discussion must be bracketed as Freke's text exists outside the framing dates and introduces concerns separate from those addressed here.

[32] Brayman Hackel, *Reading Material*; Johns, *The Nature of the Book*; Leong, "Introduction" in *Receipt Books, c. 1575–1800*; Fred Schurink, "An Elizabethan Grammar School Exercise Book," *Bodleian Library Record* 18.2 (October 2003): 174–96.

[33] Leong and Pennell, "Recipe Collections and Medical Knowledge," 133; and Field, "Writing the Self."

[34] We may counterpose the Bulckley text, for example, to the Freke manuscript, mentioned above. Leong has positioned Freke's recipe collection and herbal epitome within the recipe book genre in her dissertation "Medical Recipe Collections in Seventeenth-Century England: Knowledge, Gender and Text." Margaret Ezell has also presented on this text as a fascinating example of "domestic papers" in the National Endowment for the Humanities Summer Institute, "The Handwritten Worlds of Early Modern England" (Folger Shakespeare Library, Washington, DC, July 25–26, 2005).

of our examples from that second chapter come without biographical detail. At moments, my work here necessarily will be speculative, as the alternative would be the exclusion of the new evidence found. Given the lacunae in women's history, speculation may be all that the fragments can allow. The evidence I bring to you is sometimes as fragmentary as a few signatures on a page, but if we bring these fragments together, looking at interrelations across texts and within texts, we can begin to see patterns. These fragments are then better illumined when a letter, a history, a will, emerges. As we will see, however, even the inscriptions themselves reveal something about the context of herbal ownership and can give us clues about how and by whom the book was used.

Obviously, the most rewarding representations of herbal reading to be considered are those when this reading occurs in conjunction with biographical detail as provided by the author. When a woman engages an herbal text within the context of a consciously constructed life story, the herbal text gains specific signification. Such is the case of the women considered in the last two chapters of this study and of the example to be examined as our third case here, Lady Anne Clifford's family triptych, which she commissioned in the later years of her life (c. 1646 when she was 56) to commemorate the final achievement of the estate for which she and her mother had fought for decades. A reexamination of this well-considered portrait, likely by Jan van Belcamp, in the context of herbalism will help us to map further the terrain of *Englishwomen's Herbal Texts*. For our specific consideration, the left panel depicts the young Anne in front of shelves of books, with *The Epitome of Gerards Herball* appearing under a stack of folios on the bottom shelf.[35]

Richard Spence, telling us how Anne's mother, Margaret Clifford, lists Gerard as "an essential source" in her alchemical experiments, makes a connection between Gerard's folio and the "manuscript of alchemical extractions" from the center panel belonging to Lady Margaret.[36] Interestingly, the daughter's educational panel has a

---

[35] Jan van Belcamp, "The Great Picture," c. 1646, Abbot Hall Art Gallery, Kendal, Cumbria. An online reproduction of the triptych can be found through the W. W. Norton site, http://www.wwnorton.com/college/english/nael/17thcentury/topic_1/illustrations/imclifford.htm (accessed February 25, 2009).

Several scholars have understandably misidentified the text in question as Gerard's *Herball* itself. See, for example, Richard Spence's list of books in the portrait, *Lady Anne Clifford, Countess of Pembroke, Dorset and Montgomery (1590–1676)* (Stroud, Gloucestershire: Stutton Publishing, 1997), 190; Furdell, *Publishing and Medicine*, 98; Edith Snook, *Women, Reading, and the Cultural Politics*, 1; George C. Williamson, *Lady Anne Clifford, Countess of Dorset, Pembroke & Montgomery, 1590–1676: Her Life, Letters and Work* (East Ardsley, Yorkshire: S. R. Publishers, 1967), 342. (Brayman Hackel's important discussion of this library in *Reading Material* does not spend time on this volume.) The designation of the text in the left panel as an actual *Herball*, however, makes it seem as though the mother's alchemical distillations are the only work thus derived.

[36] Spence, *Lady Anne Clifford*, 190, 192. For an extended discussion of Margaret Clifford's manuscript, see Penny Bayer, "Lady Margaret Clifford's Alchemical Receipt

similar "extraction," *The Epitome*. In directing the painter to represent the epitome rather than the actual herbal, Clifford may be referring to the processes, not just the material, of her girlhood education. While shorter versions of Gerard's text (see Chapter 4) do make it into print, none of those listed in the *Short Title Catalogue* bear the title word "epitome" or appear in such a large volume; moreover, the inclusion of a print epitome in her library would not portray the intended image of abundance in learning and wealth, and would imply that Anne did not have access to the entire text. *The Epitome* represented in the triptych, therefore, may very well represent a work of Anne Clifford's own hand. As a girl, she may have copied out relevant passages of the herbal as she read it, and in this exercise, she echoed her mother's own writing practice evidenced in her alchemical distillations in the middle panel. In this way, the presence of the herbal reflects more directly the influence between mother and daughter so vital in Clifford's life-writings.[37] In those writings, Lady Anne constructs her relationship with her mother as one of healing; significantly, as Doreen Nagy notes, Clifford reports sending an herbal medicament to her mother in the same way she records sitting by her daughter's bedside in her fits of ague, and Clifford also registers a pride in her mother's medical practice in her later recounting of family history.[38] Regarding the epitome as a volume written in the young Anne's own hand recognizes Gerard's presence but does not give him primacy; instead, it foregrounds the education (and the maternal influence in that education) that the panel is meant to capture.

Clifford has reading the herbal portrayed alongside a family history of childhood death (the two brothers in the middle panel not having survived to adulthood) and female inheritance at the same time that she constructs the reading of the herbal as *part of* the family history. In denoting herbal knowledge and with it herbal practice in a specified context, the text represented is no longer fixed and only Gerard's. It signifies the relationship between mother and daughter as a relationship of safe-guarding the health, physical as well as economic, of the household. Of course, familial female network is part of the general myth that Clifford means to purvey for her audience in writing her autobiography and in commissioning the painting,[39] and as a result, this authorial self-construction informs how the epitome comes to take on meaning in relation to and apart from Gerard's established authority. This mythic self-construction through related texts at once draws on Gerard's name at the same time as it works to add depth and authority to Clifford's own. Women

Book and the John Dee Circle," *AMBIX* 52.3 (November 2005): 271–84.

[37] For discussions of this relationship see especially Barbara Lewalski, *Writing Women in Jacobean England* (Cambridge, Massachusetts: Harvard University Press, 1993) and Spence, *Lady Anne Clifford*.

[38] Anne Clifford, *The Memoir of 1603 and The Diary of 1616–1619*, ed. Katherine O. Acheson (Peterborough, Ontario: Broadview Editions, 2007), 41 and 115–23; Nagy, *Popular Medicine*, 13, 60, and 65; Bayer, "Lady Margaret Clifford's Alchemical Receipt Book," 276.

[39] See Lewalski, *Writing Women*, 125–52.

writing in other economic, geographic, marital, religious, and familial contexts such as those discussed in the third and fourth chapters differently displace, replace, or engage the medical authority the herbal text may otherwise represent.

In essence, the example of Clifford shows the process of differentiation that occurs when the text becomes incorporated into a specific woman's life. The abstraction of the ur-text (in itself not represented) becomes a signifier of the practical education—a kind of education that figures throughout my study here—of which it was a part, thus giving the authoritative herbal a rhetorical function particular to Clifford's family history. The writing process of distillation or epitomization, therefore, brings us to the individuation at the core of this study: the herbs a woman chooses to use, the herbal she reads, the method and the context in which she uses herbs and reads herbals, are as variable as the physiologies, biographies, and climates involved. So even though an herbal itself may attempt to paint one "Gentlewoman Reader," a woman's engagement with herbal language is in no way predetermined by that authoritative text. Those moments in which a woman claims some relationship to herbal knowledge then gain significance through their practicality in both senses of that word: in their relationship to practice and in their exclusion of that which is not directly relevant. In outlining the practices of Clifford, as well as of the Bulckley Compiler A, I am not attempting to assert a binary between epitome and authority. Rather I would prefer to see the comprehensive and the necessary as two related but separately functioning modes. In delineating these modes here, I aim to take some of the dominance out of comprehensiveness as asserted in the herbals by their male authors and to give weight to another relationship to knowledge, one that also has purpose and integrity and one that reads for immediate and personal application.[40]

Finally, the practice of epitomization points to another aspect of herbal reading that must be addressed. Namely, epitomization can be and is often linked to questions of economic access: a woman may create an epitome from a borrowed text because she cannot afford to own the expensive folio original. This economic factor comes into this study not only in the way the print epitomes of authoritative herbals discussed in Chapter 4 take on these questions directly but also in the implicit way many of the women's engagements with these texts voice overarching concerns about access to medical care. Even in Gerard's construction of "women of all sorts, especially … such as cure and helpe the poore and impotent of your countrie without rewarde" (288), we can see the necessities of charitable care, but when looking from the vantage of the "poore and impotent," we see how a more affordable and concentrated circulation of extensive herbal knowledge becomes desirable. It is in this spirit that we consider Isabella Whitney's *Sweet Nosgay*, a work that may seem separate from chapters that consider early modern gentlewomen's relationship to the authoritative herbal texts, but in its analogous engagement with less authoritative herbal works and in the author's figurative

---

[40] Cf. Elaine Leong's conception of "practical reading" in Leong, "Medical Recipe Collections in Seventeenth-Century England."

self-positioning as a poor and unemployed herbalist walking the streets of London, Whitney's text provides an important instance of diverse reading in women's herbalism. Whitney's *Nosgay*—like, in effect, every example studied in the following chapters—demonstrates yet one more signifying potential in Englishwomen's herbal texts and points to further possibilities beyond our focus here.

Chapter 1
"This Manlike Worke of Herbes": Gender and the English Herbal

In John Gerard's *Herball*, the last entry under the virtues "Of water Dockes"—sometimes called "bastarde rubarbe," "garden Patience," or "bloudwort"—is a long one. In establishing the efficacy of the herbs in helping patients to "cure" the ague, Gerard cites not only his own experience but also the results of the "notable experiment" of "one *Iohn Bennet*, a chirurgion of Maidstone in Kent," a man whom he calls "as slenderly learned as my selfe." After relating Bennet's "blunt" (though successful) "attempt" at finding a cure, Gerard expresses the hope that Bennet's coarse success may motivate those with "greater iudgement in the faculties of plants, to seeke farther into their nature then any of the auncients haue done: and none fitter then the learned phisitions of the Colledge of London; where are many singularly well learned, and experienced in naturall things."[1]

Gerard's account of the success of surgeons and his subsequent challenge to the other "tripartite" members of the college would seem to be a classic example of competition in the medical market, except that the entry has not yet finished. In a short paragraph separate from the long one recounting Bennet's experiment (yet still part of the same virtue description), Gerard tells his reader, "The rootes sliced and boiled in the water of Carduus Benedictus . . . adding thereto a little honie, of the which decoction eight or ten sponfuls drunke before the fit, cureth the ague in two or three times [of] taking it at the most" (315). Neither surgeon nor physician came up with this cure, however; Gerard provides the following attribution: "This experiment was practiced by a worshipfull gentlewoman called mistress *Anne Wylbraham*, vpon diuers of hir poore neighbours with good successe" (315). Outside of royal patrons, archetypal wisewoman, and classical precedent (all of which will be discussed below), Anne Wilbraham is the only actual woman to be named within any English authoritative herbal before 1650, and this distinction would seem to make her exemplary. Her work stands alongside that of surgeons and physicians, and her name balances that of John Bennet in the text. In this way, Gerard affirms her role as medical experimenter, makes her known as one of his practitioner compatriots, and folds her into the establishment of herbal authority.

Describing Wilbraham as a gentlewoman who administers to "her poor neighbors," Gerard contributes to the constructions of the gentlewoman reader in the text, who stands opposed to "the beggerly rabble of witches, charmers, &

---

[1] John Gerard, *The Herball or Generall Historie of Plantes* (London, 1597), 312–15. Subsequent citations included in the text.

such like couseners, that regarde more to get money then to helpe for charitie" (288) seen in Gerard's entry on tobacco discussed in our introduction. In depicting Wilbraham's work as charitable, he sets the parameters for female medical experiment. In naming Wilbraham, he introduces another family of influence with whom he was acquainted and into which Anne Pierson married in 1586, the Wilbrahams of Nantwich.[2] In relating Wilbraham's success, Gerard not only provides a model for his female readership, he may also present a challenge to find cures to that readership in the way he delivers one to the College of Physicians. In thus targeting his female audience, he acknowledges a broad base of female practitioners who may encounter his text, but again, in naming even one woman experimenter, he is the exception in the establishment of the English tradition before 1650.

This chapter considers how and to what ends the English authoritative herbal tradition represented the female herbal practitioner in her various guises. In doing so it asks how the English tradition may have established its medical authority by seeking to limit and exclude those women who practiced to "get money" at the same time that it affirmed, defined, and contained the gentlewoman reader/practitioner. While Gerard's mention is the only named nonroyal female practitioner, there are other unnamed or pseudonymously named women who handled herbs represented in the texts. That many of them may have been categorized among the "beggerly rabble of witches" delineated by Gerard shows us much about the anxieties in the establishment of the herbal tradition. As we will see, the authorial anxiety in herbal texts stemmed in part from the fact that practitioners existed who preceded textual authority. What is more, the authors could no more have controlled the use of the text than they could have stopped a woman from copying its pages. Thus representing the desired yet uncontrollable female practitioner became a part of the generic conventions of the authoritative English herbal.

The dates framing this study, 1550–1650, roughly coincide with the establishment of this textual tradition with its sets of conventions and anti-conventions not yet catalogued by literary historians. While cultural historians such as Mary Fissell have begun to examine works of vernacular medicine as indicators of social change and Rebecca Bushnell and Jennifer Munroe have provided us with in-depth assessments of gardening manuals from the period, literary historians are only beginning to articulate the tropes and themes of the vernacular herbal tradition.[3] A feminist analysis of the herbals' tropes and themes, especially at this moment when feminist criticism is considering alternative narratives to that of

---

2 Robert H. Jeffers, *The Friends of John Gerard (1545–1612): Surgeon and Botanist* (Falls Village, Connecticut: The Herb Grower Press, 1967), 61.

3 Mary E. Fissell, *Vernacular Bodies: The Politics of Reproduction in Early Modern England* (Oxford: Oxford University Press, 2004); Rebecca W. Bushnell, *Green Desire: Imagining Early Modern English Gardens* (Ithaca, New York: Cornell University Press, 2003); and Jennifer Munroe, *Gender and the Garden in Early Modern English Literature* (Burlington, Vermont: Ashgate Publishing, 2008). A recent literary analysis of this tradition

the subjugation of women, will help us to distinguish between the rhetorical and historical realities of early modern medicine. Even though the medical practice of certain women—i.e., gentlewomen—may be informed by the rhetoric of the herbals that looks to limit irregular practice as part of the "aim of minority groups" to establish a system of control run by physicians, surgeons, apothecaries, as discussed in the introduction,[4] an alternative reading of the gendered language in these texts considers how this language tells us more about anxieties surrounding the formation of the tradition in English—a tradition that had arrived belatedly to the British Isles and had recently been infused with New World plants and practices—than about actual practice. As with the sonnet sequence, England was late in contributing to a textual tradition already well established on the Continent, and some of its best-known contributions to the tradition could be seen as simply translations of continental texts. This late entry into the field colors the pages of the early herbal texts just as the prior presence of Petrarch and Ronsard casts a shadow on the sonnets of Wyatt, Surrey, and Sidney.

Early twentieth-century herbal historians Eleanour Rohde and Agnes Arber place the beginning of a distinctively English herbal tradition between the first work (1551) of William Turner, known as "the Father of British Botany,"[5] and the *Theatrum Botanicum* (1640) of John Parkinson, "[t]he last of the great English herbalists."[6] In surveying this early stage of the tradition, this chapter considers the herbals of Turner, Rembert Dodoens (as translated by Henry Lyte), Gerard (arguably the most popular of the herbalists), and Parkinson. I have limited the discussion in this chapter to these authors' herbals as they have four aspects in common: they claim authority, work toward comprehensiveness, appear in print, and are written in English.

All four authors lay claim to extensive knowledge of their precursors, both ancient and continental, thus revealing their erudition. The prefatory materials and individual entries refer to ancient Greek and Roman authorities such as Pliny the

---

can be found in Leah Knight, *Of Books and Botany in Early Modern England* (Burlington, Vermont: Ashgate Publishing, 2009).

4 Margaret Pelling, "Trade or Profession?: Medical Practice in Early Modern England," *The Common Lot: Sickness, Medical Occupations and the Urban Poor in Early Modern England* (Harlow, Essex: Longman, 1998), 244.

5 Seeming to glean the title from Benjamin Daydon Jackson's biography included in the same volume, William Thomas Stearn relates how Turner "earned from posterity his title as the 'Father of British Botany'" in his edition of Turner's *Libellus de Re Herbaria, 1538, [and] The Name of Herbes, 1548* (London: Ray Society, 1965), ix and 15. Agnes Arber also repeats the title from Jackson's biography; Agnes Arber, *Herbals, their Origin and Evolution: A Chapter in the History of Botany, 1470–1670* (1912; reprint, Cambridge: Cambridge University Press, 1953), 119. See also S. E. B., "An Elizabethan Herbal," *More Books: A Bulletin of the Boston Public Library* 25 (1940): 245.

6 Eleanour Sinclair Rohde, *The Old English Herbals* (1922; reprint, New York: Dover Publications, Inc., 1971), 142; Arber, *Herbals*. See also Blanche Henrey, *British Botanical and Horticultural Literature before 1800* (London: Oxford University Press, 1975).

Elder (C. E. 23–79), Dioscorides (C. E. 40–90), and Galen (C. E. 129–216) and authorities in Arabic such as Averroës (C. E. 1126–1198/1206). Turner's work is most overt about this relationship to his ancient and medieval sources, with some of his entries on plants including subheadings that read "Out of Plinie" or "Oute of Galene."[7] Unlike other vernacular volumes, however, these herbals are not merely English translations or derivatives of ancient manuscripts but seek to synthesize the knowledge before them. Thus English herbal entries also incorporate the arguments and experiments of continental counterparts, which include the French translations of Jean Ruel (1516)[8] and Charles de L'Écluse (1554) and similar Latin and vernacular synthesizing projects of Hieronymus Bock (1546), Otto Brunfels (1530, 1531, 1540), and Leonhart Fuchs (1542) of Germany, Pietro Andrea Mattioli (1544) of Italy, Dodoens (1554) of the Spanish Lowlands, and the Latin contributions by Pierre Pena of France and Matthias de l'Obel of Flanders (1570), as well as the description of colonial plants by Nicolás Monardes (1569).[9] As we will see below, Turner, being the earliest of the English compilers, has a much more fraught relationship with his German, Flemish, and Italian counterparts, but his consolation could be that he would become a resource for subsequent English herbals as well as others written and revised on the Continent. In the 1633 version of Gerard's herbal, editor Thomas Johnson cites all of the above, including Turner, Lyte, and Parkinson, and of course Gerard, as crucial pieces in the long tradition before him. Of course, for our feminist purposes, it is important to point out that in the English authoritative textual tradition, no woman has a substantial role. While post-second-wave feminist scholars such as Frank Anderson include the work of Hildegard of Bingen in their description of the European tradition, the English authors, most dramatically seen in Johnson's articulation of his herbal progenitors, claimed a male-only lineage.[10]

The second trait these herbals share is that they claim to approach comprehensiveness. Indicative of this trait is the language of enlargement, sometimes in conjunction with the word "all," in the extended titles of these works. That the 1568 edition of *The first and seconde partes of the Herbal of William Turner* is "corrected and enlarged with the Thirde parte" demonstrates that Turner's life work strives toward a more complete picture of the names and traits of herbs. Dodoens's *Nievve Herball, or Historie of Plantes* purports to "contain"

---

[7] William Turner, *The first and seconde partes of the Herbal of William Turner Doctor in Phisick / lately ouersene / corrected and enlarged with the Thirde parte / lately gathered* (Cologne, 1568), e.g., 1.14 and 1.166. Subsequent citations included in the text.

[8] Dates in parentheses indicate those of earliest publications.

[9] See Arber, *Herbals*, for further bibliographical information on Continental volumes.

[10] Frank J. Anderson, *An Illustrated History of the Herbals* (New York: Columbia University Press, 1977). The only exception is the figure of Artemisia. See Appendix A for a discussion of how this ancient queen becomes an important personage in the formation of the English tradition in particular but not necessarily for her role in herbalism.

"the vvhole discourse and perfect description of all sortes of Herbes and Plantes."[11] Gerard's 1597 *Herball or Generall Historie of Plantes* includes new plants such as the potato, with which Gerard is famously pictured at the end of the front matter, as well as other plants of the "New World," and is later "very much enlarged and amended" by Johnson in 1633.[12] Finally, and this is a point to come back to in our discussion of gender in these texts, the second title page of Parkinson's *Theatrum Botanicum*, the longest of the works, sells the text as:

> An herball of a large extent: Containing therein a more ample and exact history and declaration of the Physicall Herbs and Plants that are in other Authours, encreased by the accesse of many hundreds of nevv, rare, and strange Plants from all the parts of the vvorld, vvith sundry Gummes, and other Physicall materials, than hath beene hitherto published by any before; And a most large demonstration of their Natures and Vertues.[13]

The largeness of the volume speaks to its comprehensiveness, a comprehensiveness that the other authors could only attempt to approach, and marks a sense of competition in the later herbalists.

The fact that all of these works appeared in print might go without saying given the nature of this chapter, but it is an important distinction in the history of the herbal, especially given numerous herbal manuscripts in the Middle Ages, most of which, however, simply transcribed or translated classical texts.[14] In print, the herbal solidifies its conventional format, one that first describes the herb and its growing conditions and then provides a list of its medicinal, and sometimes culinary and cosmetic, aspects. Developments within these conventions as seen, for example, in Gerard's system of indexing, which labels each virtue with a different letter, contribute to the popularity of individual herbals. The importance of print

---

11 Rembert Dodoens, *A Nievve Herball, or Historie of Plantes*, trans. Henry Lyte (London, 1578).

12 John Gerard, *The Herball or Generall Historie of Plantes, Gathered by Iohn Gerard of London Master in Chirurgerie, Very much Enlarged and Amended by Thomas Iohnson* (London, 1633).

13 John Parkinson, *Theatrum Botanicum, the Theater of Plantes* (London, 1640), second title page.

14 See Rohde, *Old English Herbals*, Arber, *Herbals*, and Henrey, *Botanical and Horticultural Literature*, for full accounts of the pre-Turner English print herbals. The essay collection edited by Jean A. Givens, Karen M. Reeds, and Alain Touwaide, *Visualizing Medieval Medicine, 1200–1500* (Burlington, Vermont: Ashgate Publishing, 2006), provides an exemplary account of scholarship on herbals in manuscript before the sixteenth century. For work on medieval manuscript herbals in England, see the following articles and other works by these scholars: George R. Keiser, "Through a Fourteenth-Century Gardener's Eyes: Henry Daniel's Herbal," *Chaucer Review: A Journal of Medieval Studies and Literary Criticism* 31.1 (1996): 58–75, and Rossell Hope Robbins, "Medical Manuscripts in Middle English," *Speculum* 45.3 (July 1970): 393–415.

in establishing this group as foundational to the tradition, however, becomes most apparent when we consider the example of Gerard's text, which has as its foundation a manuscript translation of Dodoens's Latin treatise *Pemptades Sex* (1583). According to Johnson, a Dr. Priest, physician, left the manuscript to his friend Gerard upon his death, and Gerard completed and revised the work, with the input of Matthias de l'Obel (living in England), a history that is also hinted at in 1597. The consequence of print in the English herbal tradition has meant that the volume is now known as Gerard's herbal, not as Priest's, and contributions to and articulations of the tradition hereafter come to recognize Turner, Dodoens, Gerard, and Parkinson as key contributors to the formation of the English herbal.

The aspect of print most relevant here, however, is how the new technology makes the herbal knowledge accessible to a general buying public and, when this accessibility is combined with the herbals' being written in English, separates the British tradition from its classical and continental counterparts. In the end, the fact that the authors write their herbals in English becomes a constitutive aspect of the works, as each must transform the tradition before them while negotiating with the detractors against their product. As Eleanour Rohde has shown us, other herbals were printed in English before Turner, but these are the first to claim to be authoritative and comprehensive. Conceivably, this combination—authoritative and comprehensive, in print and in English—gives the reader of the English herbal—in theory the male professional but in practice including the (often female) layperson—access to almost as much herbal knowledge as the "learned physician," which, as we will see, becomes a point of anxiety for author and physician alike.

At the same time that they provided this access, the folio volumes of Turner, Lyte, Gerard, and Parkinson also did their part in the gendering of medical–textual authority in early modern England. Not only did they provide witness to the changing face of medical practice in that time and place; they contributed to it. Medical historians have described the increase in the regulation of medical practice after the establishment of the College of Physicians (1518) and the 1542 act that allowed unlicensed practitioners only if they administered medicine without asking for payment.[15] It would *seem* that, at least in London, legitimate practice was thus relegated to the positions of physician, surgeon, and apothecary, but as previously discussed, Margaret Pelling and others have noted that "medical practice in early modern England was neither well organised nor firmly controlled."[16] The prefatory materials of authoritative vernacular print herbals from 1550 to 1650—even the individual plant entries—were informed by and consequently contributed to the status and gender prejudices and repressive hierarchies found in the "tripartite

[15] For example, see Andrew Wear, *Knowledge and Practice in English Medicine, 1550–1680* (Cambridge: Cambridge University Press, 2000), and Margaret Pelling (with Frances White), *Medical Conflicts in Early Modern London: Patronage, Physicians, and Irregular Practitioners, 1550–1640* (Oxford: Clarendon Press, 2003).

[16] Pelling, "Trade or Profession?" 244.

structure" of practice, marking some of the herbalists members of the "minority groups" who kept it their "aim" to establish and maintain that structure.[17]

The gendering of medical authority in these volumes depends upon a hierarchy that puts male educated textual knowledge above female, most often uneducated, practical knowledge; thus both male and female practitioners are represented in the establishment of that medical authority. In this respect, my analysis also bears some relation to Londa Schiebinger's discussion of the iconographic representations of women within scientific discourse in the seventeenth and eighteenth centuries. Schiebinger explores the removal of women from scientific practice and the coinciding framing of scientific debates in gendered terms, most glaringly in the writings of Francis Bacon.[18] These scientific writings remove women in theory if not in actuality, and in the individual—sometimes proto-Baconian—examples examined here, the seemingly random—sometimes contradictory—appearances of women as keepers and purveyors of herbal knowledge reflect the tensions and inconsistencies within the gendered constructs of the herbal tradition and, by extension, medical authority in early modern England. The fact that the women represented are from all economic strata is indicative of both the contradictions in and the motivations behind these representations.

So while it is well established that women practiced herbalism and that they did so before and after the publication of these treatises, and while the herbal texts look to account for and control that practice, my study is more pointedly concerned with the ways in which the domination of a largely male textual medical authority over predominantly female traditional practical knowledge is represented in these texts for reasons other than the historical subjugation of women. When female herbal authorities appear in male-authored English herbal texts, they signify beyond their known existence in historical reality and become the figures onto which the authors of these herbal texts may displace anxieties about their own herbal textual project. Specifically, these figures come to bear the onus for errors in male authoritative texts, rivalries within the English tradition, any misapplications in self/other-medication the texts may facilitate, and even the gendered political tensions surrounding publication. These herbals accomplish this displacement through the division of herbal knowledge into unstable and gendered binaries, through long-standing mythic structures of dominance, and through the rhetorical restriction of female power to domestic categories. Such maneuvers in the texts bear witness to the living presence of female herbal authority, but they also betray the inconsistencies and tensions found in the male herbal textual tradition.

---

17 Pelling, "Trade or Profession?" 244.

18 Londa Schiebinger, *The Mind Has No Sex? Women in the Origins of Modern Science* (Cambridge, Massachusetts: Harvard University Press, 1989), 137–38.

Gendering the English Herbal

In the dedication of his *Theatrum Botanicum* (1640), John Parkinson, "Apothecary of London and the Kings Herbarist," describes his 1,755-page treatise on plants and their medicinal uses as "this Manlike Worke of Herbes and Plants."[19] In this phrase, Parkinson may refer to any of a number of the herbal's features. Based on the perceived "robust physique" of the Renaissance man,[20] he may make a physical correlation; the alternatively titled "an herball of a large extent," weighs eleven pounds. He may allude to the "long paines and endeavours" he took in "compos[ing]" the *Theatrum*, eleven years from the publication of his *Paradisi in Sole Paradisus Terrestris* (1629); his work is thus "manlike" in its Herculean or Odyssean aspect.[21] He finally may provide a more direct hint in the contradistinction he makes to that earlier work, which he calls "a Feminine of Flowers" in the *Theatrum* dedication; "herbes" are a more medicinally specific category, thus referring to the male domination of institutional medicine—physicians, surgeons, and apothecaries—in the period.[22] As a result, this gendering may show Parkinson's position as a member of one of the "minority groups" named by Pelling, whose main goal was the control of medical practice by this "tripartite structure in England."[23] As part of this gendering of subject matter, Parkinson may also be gendering his readership; where the implicit, often overt, reader in the first volume is female (with occasional nods to the professional male gardener),[24] the represented reader of the *Theatrum* is decidedly male. All of these—size, extent, subject, and readership—point to ways in which the volume could be *perceived* to be masculine. They do not, however, account for the need to name it so. By what means and for what reasons the "worke of herbes" comes to be called "manlike" is the central question of this section.

In part, Parkinson follows the lead of English herbalists before him and asserts the volume's "manlike" qualities in part to counteract associations that exist outside the text that connect herbal practice with women and household labors. My understanding here builds upon Pelling's reading of the "insecurities of status" felt by English physicians of the early modern period. Pelling writes that "wherever men appropriated tasks associated with women or with feminized spaces within the household, they incurred some penalty in status terms."[25] Given the overlap between the subject of the educated herbalists and the occupations of

19 Parkinson, "To the Kings Most Excellent Maiestie," *Theatrum Botanicum*, n. p.

20 Ian Maclean, *The Renaissance Notion of Woman: A Study in the Fortunes of Scholasticism and Medical Science in European Intellectual Life* (Cambridge: Cambridge University Press, 1980), 46.

21 Parkinson, "To the Kings Most Excellent Maiestie," *Theatrum Botanicum*, n. p.

22 Parkinson, "To the Kings Most Excellent Maiestie," *Theatrum Botanicum*, n. p.

23 Pelling, "Trade or Profession?" 244.

24 Bushnell, *Green Desire*.

25 Pelling, *Medical Conflicts in Early Modern London*, 191.

the illiterate herbwife, the wisewoman/witch, and the gentlewoman practitioner (all of whom are considered in this chapter), herbal texts reveal similar insecurities about the status and gender associations of the work they represent. I suggest that these "insecurities of status" only in part account for this treatment of female practitioners; much of this chapter works to uncover other sources of herbal authorial anxiety and demonstrate how these "insecurities" also come forward in rhetorical moves that are notably inflected by gender.

Even though Parkinson's text seems most loaded with insecurity, before discussing his texts in depth I will first examine the herbals of William Turner, whose designation as the "Father of British Botany" will soon resonate more profoundly for us.[26] His *New Herball* (1551) is seen to be the first truly English foray into the herbal genre. Those herbals printed before his in England, namely *Bancke's Herbal* (1525) and the *Grete Herball* (1526), though interesting in their own right, are not infused with issues of textual authority that we find in Turner and post-Turner publications.[27] Turner's three volumes, from 1551, 1562, 1568, all concern themselves with the newness of the task he assumes, that is, to produce in English the names and uses of English herbs, both those included in the works of the ancients and those not so. Turner's two small works that precede these in 1538 and 1548 (*Libellus de Re Herbaria* and *The Names of Herbs*) anticipate this task in undertaking the cataloging of those herbs, first in Latin then in English. A physician and Protestant minister, Turner mainly gleans his authority from his education at Oxford and his fieldwork in Germany and Italy, the latter of which was forced exploration, as he was exiled for nonconformity during the reigns of Henry VIII and Mary. His approach shows keen awareness of the textual authorities that precede him while drawing on his continental experience.

The rhetorical moves of Turner's prefaces, however, also reveal his acute anxieties about the nature of his work, especially in its dependence on continental precursors and its association with female practitioners. In his dedication to Queen Elizabeth I from the 1568 folio that contains the first, second, and third volumes of his work, Turner imagines critics who would accuse him of "mak[ing] . . . frendes with other mennis trauayles,"[28] in other words, of merely replicating the work of his ancient and continental sources and presenting it to the queen as his own. Turner is thus determined in his questioning of the textual authorities that have been "set oute" (*3r) in the sixteenth century. With no pretense of modesty, he tells his sovereign how he "dyd frendlie admonishe [Leonhart Fuchs] of certeyne erroures that were in his herball" and "borrowed verye littel or ellis nothinge of Matthiolus" (*3r); he does so in order to refute his anticipated critics but also to establish his own authority by showing the errors of his continental counterparts:

---

[26] See n. 5, above.

[27] See Rohde, *Old English Herbals*, 55–74.

[28] William Turner, *The first and seconde partes of the Herbal*, *3r. Subsequent citations included in the text. Virgules are from the original text and stand in lieu of punctuation.

> they that haue red the first part of my Herbal / & haue compared my writinges of plantes with those thinges that Matthiolus / Fuchsius / Tragus [Bock] / and Dodoneus wrote in ye firste editiones of their Herballes / maye easely perceyue that I taught the truthe of certeyne plantes / which these aboue named writers either knew not at al / or ellis erred in thē greatlye. (*3r)

For the first part of the dedication the source of error lies on the Continent.

When Turner then similarly compares "many Physiciones" "lyke unto a cryer y^{t} cryeth a loste horse in the marketh [*sic*] / & telleth all the markes and tokens that he hath / & yet neuer sawe the horse" (sig. *3r), it would at first seem that he equates the practice of physicians with those herbalists who do not check their textual sources through experiment. As the analogy develops, however, this critique of written and learned authority slides into suspicion of the unlearned sources behind such authority:

> I wente into Italye and into diuerse partes of Germany / to knowe and se the herbes my self / and to knowe by practise their powers and workinge / not trustinge onlye to the olde herbe wiues and apothecaryes (as manye Physiciones haue done of late yeres) but in the mater of simples myne / owne eyes and knowledge. (sig. *3r)

In Turner's analogy, the source of the mistakes in contemporary texts and practice is not the replication of other texts but in an overdependence on *illiterate*, or Latin-illiterate sources, on "herbe wives," women who collected plant materials for physicians and apothecaries, and the apothecaries themselves. As the passage earlier in the preface makes clear, however, it is textual knowledge that has proven unreliable, and Turner attempts here to displace this unreliability onto the very individuals who do not have access to that textual knowledge. The introduction of the herbwives and apothecaries creates scapegoats for all transmission of unreliable herbal knowledge. In such a figuration, the herbwives and apothecaries become prototypes for Spenser's Error, the tail of which includes a long history of mistranslation and unverified assertions. Paradoxically, the specter of textual fallibility is embodied through figures that have no relation to texts. As depicted in the herbal, the herbwife and the apothecary transmit their knowledge orally. In true proto-Spenserian fashion, moreover, this figure in the end becomes decidedly female.[29]

---

29 This insight also leads us to the question, in part spurred by the coney-catching version of the "loste horse" scenario in which the con-man is responsible for both stealing and recovering the horse, of whether or not the "horse" was ever lost at all, and if so, who was responsible for losing it. Samuel Rid, "The Art of Juggling or Legerdemain" (1612), in *Rogues, Vagabonds, & Sturdy Beggars*, ed. Arthur F. Kinney (Amherst: University of Massachusetts Press, 1990), 280.

The insight that illiterate figures may be standing in for errors made by scholars relates to the suggestive analysis conducted by Steven Shapin of scientific discourse in the seventeenth century, in which "unreliable testimony was routinely labeled as 'old wives tales.'"[30] Turner thus creates a hierarchy of learned physicians such as himself at the top, learned-but-somewhat-uncareful herbalists/physicians and dark doctors/unlearned physicians below, and apothecaries and herbwives at the bottom. He purports that he revises this hierarchy, however, through the herbal, which is

> necessarye for Phisiciones & apothecaries w^t^out ye knowlege whereof they can not deuly [*sic*] exercise their office and vocation where vnto they are called / for howe can he be a good artificer that neither knoweth the names of hys toles / nether the toles themselfes when he seeth. (sig. *3r)

Turner here seems to be repeating the sentiments of the lost-horse passage with artisan imagery, but the names of the players have changed. Whereas before the physician did not know the "lost horse," i.e., herbs, and thus was too dependent on the "olde herbe wiues and apothecaryes," here within the same paragraph, the physicians *and apothecaries* learn to recognize and name the "tools" of their trade through the herbal. Through the vernacular text and their knowledge of written English, the apothecaries are divorced from the herbwomen and are united with the physicians. Turner thus displaces the illiterate and female bottom of the hierarchy and with it an unreliable herbal tradition.

If we return to the source of his analogy, however, it is clear that the herbwife, or any other woman involved with plants for that matter, has not been responsible for the loss of true herbal knowledge. On the contrary, in the analogy, Turner reveals that she may be one of the few remaining preservers of that knowledge. Yes, Turner probably follows the lead of one of his continental sources, Leonhart Fuchs, and before him Pliny (who does not gender this ignorance), but he revises Fuchs's contention.[31] Also, with these other herbalists, Turner may also imitate, like early astronomers Galileo and Kepler, "patristic writers" for whom "old wives' tales were associated with the various pagan myths and hermeneutic

---

[30] Steven Shapin, *A Social History of Truth: Civility and Science in Seventeenth-Century England* (Chicago: The University of Chicago Press, 1994), 90.

[31] In his letter to Joachim II, margrave of Brandenburg, Fuchs blames physicians for leaving "plant investigation" to "the drug sellers . . . and to stupid and frightfully superstitious old wives. So much so that the whole field of herbal medicine is in the hands of rustic and decrepit old women and illiterate people, who heap error upon error." Leonhart Fuchs, *The Great Herbal of Leonhart Fuchs: De Historia Stirpium Commentarii Insignes, 1542 (Notable Commentaries on the History of Plants)*, ed. and trans. Frederick G. Meyer, Emily Emmart Trueblood, and John L. Heller (Stanford: Stanford University Press, 1999), 204, and Pliny the Elder, *Natural History*, trans., W. H. S. Jones (Cambridge, Massachusetts: Harvard University Press, 1956), XXV.vi.

practices against which the early church . . . defined itself," as Eileen Reeves has so deftly illustrated, in making old wives stand in for all "crude and unthinking supporters" of superstitious and unfounded beliefs.[32] Iconographically, the "old wife" in England becomes the wisewoman/witch at the fringes of culture. In Turner's herbal, however, the holders of herbal knowledge are not only "old wives" and "drug sellers"[33] but also Fuchs, Mattioli, and Bock. Ironically, what Turner's text attempts to accomplish is the de-feminization of herbal knowledge while at the same time dispersing anxieties about the unreliability of the classical and continental *textual* tradition and current licensed medical practice. As Turner's text rhetorically removes the herbwife from the circle of medical practice, it expunges with her any misgivings about the errors of previous practice and texts and about the belated English presence in the print herbal tradition.

Even though Turner's herbwife may in part register the living presence of actual sellers of herbs in the marketplace—a living presence rarely found in archival work[34]—her presence in this text may be more significant in exposing the anxieties about and complications in the gendering of medical authority. While the result of Turner's rhetoric may be the exclusion of the herbwife from further discussions of herbal authority, similar anxieties and complications return throughout the establishment of the English herbal tradition and do so in pointedly gendered terms. The authorial example that begins this section and a much later contributor to the tradition, Parkinson, similarly uses female figures to take on the history of lost or suspect herbal knowledge as he overtly genders his herbal project.

Parkinson masculinizes the herbal tradition, the "Manlike Worke of Herbes," in two stages: first, through the feminization of his *Paradisus Terrestris*, then through the hyper-masculinization of his *Theatrum Botanicum*. At first, however, it would seem that the earlier work strives for gender parity. The frontispiece of the *Paradisus*, presumably not designed by Parkinson, represents an ornate Garden of Eden in which a naked Adam and Eve combine their efforts in the collection and propagation of plants (Figure 1.1). The image is proto-baroque in its execution; the lines are a combination of feminine curves and snake-like vines crossed by straight and enormous trees (most iconographically identified with the phallus as one grows virtually from Adam's groin). This seeming equality dissolves, however, with Parkinson's address to his reader, with the written word. In the following passage and its allusion to Genesis, Parkinson makes an argument for the rightful

[32] Eileen Reeves, "Old Wives Tales and the New World System," *Configurations* 7.3 (Fall 1999): 303.

[33] Fuchs, *The Great Herbal*, 204.

[34] The exceptions here are brief citations by Deborah E. Harkness, "'Strange' Ideas and 'English' Knowledge: Natural Science Exchange in Elizabethan London," in *Merchants and Marvels: Commerce, Science, and Art in Early Modern Europe*, ed. Pamela H. Smith and Paula Findlen (New York: Routledge, 2002), 144–45, and Doreen Evenden Nagy, *Popular Medicine in Seventeenth-Century England* (Bowling Green, Ohio: Bowling Green State University Popular Press, 1988), 78.

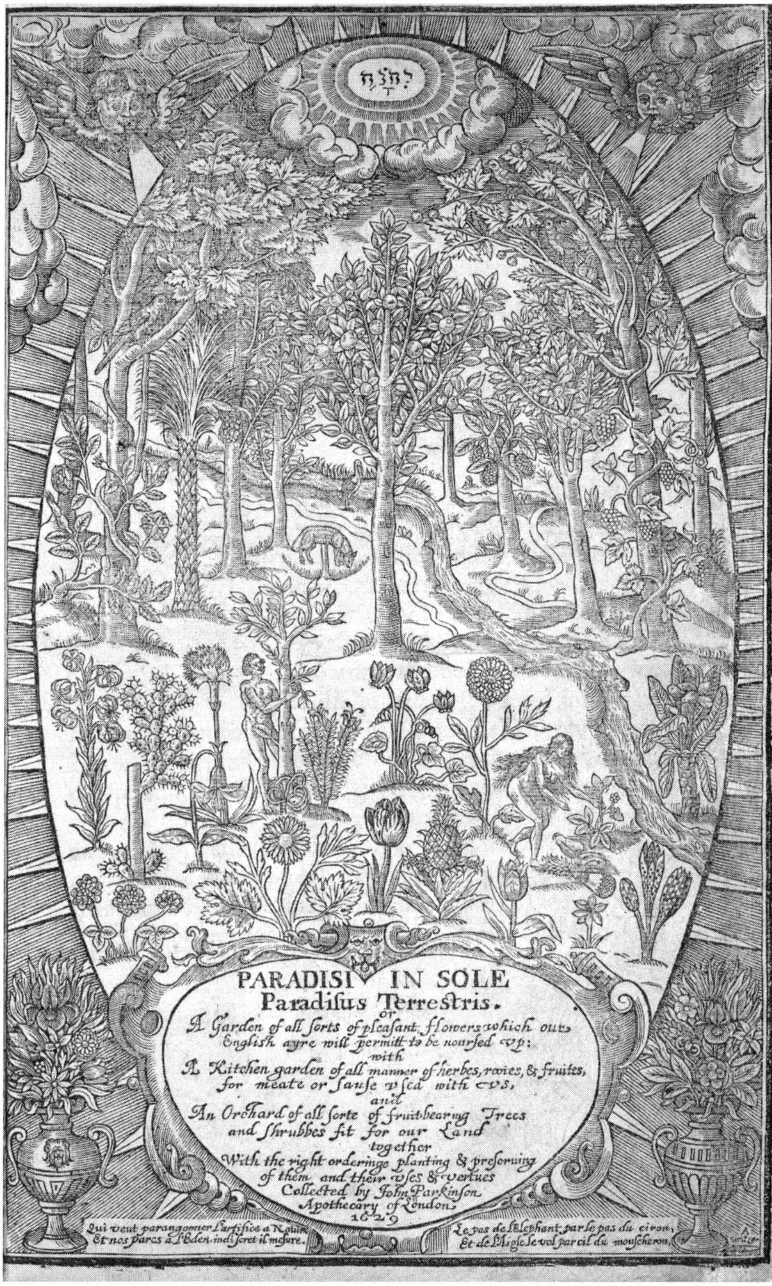
PARADISI IN SOLE
Paradisus Terrestris.
or
A Garden of all sorts of pleasant flowers which our
English ayre will permitt to be noursed vp:
with
A Kitchen garden of all manner of herbes, rootes, & fruites,
for meate or sause vsed with vs,
and
An Orchard of all sorte of fruitbearing Trees
and shrubbes fit for our Land
together
With the right orderinge planting & preseruing
of them and their vses & vertues
Collected by John Parkinson
Apothecary of London
1629
Qui veut parangonner l'artifice a Nature
Et nos parcs a l'Eden indiscret il mesure.
Le pas de l'elephant par le pas du ciron,
Et de l'Aigle le vol par cil du mouscheron,

Fig. 1.1 Frontispiece from John Parkinson's *Paradisi in Sole Paradisus Terrestris* (1629). Courtesy of the Library of Congress.

attainment by men (and, as made clear earlier in the preface, specifically *Judeo-Christian* men) of herbal authority:

> And although *Adam* lost the place for this transgression, yet he lost not the naturall knowledge, nor vse of them . . . Let men therefore according to their first institution, so vse their seruice, that they also in them may remember their seruice to God, and not (like our Grand-mother *Eve*) set their affections so strongly on the pleasure in them, as to deserue the losse of them . . . .[35]

The "them" here refers to the "trees and herbes" to which Adam "was able to giue names" and about which "hee had . . . the knowledge, both what Herbes and Fruits were fit, eyther for Meate or Medicine, for Vse or for Delight" (sig. ***3r). It is perhaps too obvious to point out that Adam, the male element who can name and codify, is responsible for the preservation of herbal knowledge, while "Grand-mother Eve," the old wife, is the one blamed for any loss that occurs. Parkinson at once creates an analogy between Adam and the herbal compiler—both being those "able to give names" and describe uses—and, in a way similar to how Turner's herbwife is removed from medical hierarchies, dismisses any practical knowledge held by women. While Turner's herbwife takes on the errors of male text and practice, Parkinson's Eve seems to carry the stigma of herbal misuse, "affections" that focus too much on sensual experience.

Although Parkinson condemns the female tradition—notoriously represented by Eve—because of its purported emphasis on pleasure, he makes his first publication one that is largely dedicated to that pleasure. The *Paradisus* is "first offered into" the "hands" of Queen Henrietta Maria, who "so much delighted with all the faire Flowers of a Garden" (the "flowers" here in part representing all of the artistic recipients of her patronage).[36] The volume begins with and is dominated by "the ordering of the Garden of Pleasure," the "pleasure" that was held too "strongly" in Eve's "affections" (sig. ***3r) and "The Garden of pleasant . . . Flowers" (sig. 5r *et passim*). What is more, as Bushnell has pointed out, even though it includes a section plainly entitled "The Ordering of the Kitchen Garden" (461), the volume itself de-emphasizes the medicinal "uses" of herbs.[37] Even though

---

35 John Parkinson, *Paradisi in Sole Paradisus Terrestris* (London, 1629), sig. ***3r. Subsequent references included in the text.

36 Parkinson, *Paradisus*, sig. **2r. For a reassessment of Queen Henrietta Maria's "cultural influence," see Melinda Gough's essay "'Not as Myself': The Queen's Voice in *Tempe Restored*," *Modern Philology* 101.1 (August 2003): 48–67. Later, after Charles I's death, the queen will come to be known for her collection of recipes, many of which were medical, called *The Queens Closet Opened* (1658), a work discussed by Lynette Hunter, "Women and Domestic Medicine: Lady Experimenters, 1570–1620," *Women, Science and Medicine 1500–1700: Mothers and Sisters of the Royal Society*, ed. Lynette Hunter and Sarah Hutton (Stroud, Gloucestershire: Sutton Publishing, 1997), 89–107.

37 Bushnell, *Green Desire*, 61–62.

some minor applications are given, the list of virtues of each garden flower and kitchen herb in *Paradisus* is but a small fraction of the same given in Parkinson's later "manlike" work. Additionally, the virtues that are given tend to concentrate on household applications—those of cooking, cleaning, and dyeing—and the cosmetic values of the plants. For example, "the leaues of the *Cortusa* taste a little hot, and if one of them bee laide whole, without bruising, on the cheeke of any tender skind woman, it will raise an orient red colour, as if some *fucus* [cosmetic] had been laide thereon, which will passe away without any manner of harme, or marke where it lay" (*Paradisus* 241). The entry for the same plant in Parkinson's *Theatrum* (534) has no such mention. In first publishing a text that concentrates on the "delights" to be found in plants and feminizing that text through its dedication and the printer's ornate frontispiece, Parkinson anticipates his second volume in which the knowledge of medicinal "uses" of plants may be masculinized and thus differentiated from knowledge necessary in household and female practice.[38]

It is important to consider the product that Parkinson sells in the *Paradisus* and to whom he sells it. Linda Levy Peck has placed it in the center of a growing sense of leisure in early modern England, and indeed, the Folger copy discussed in Chapter 2, which contains random examples of painting in the illustrations, in part supports this positioning of the text. The "Garden of Pleasure" in particular points to the future of gardening as a pastime over a simple utilitarian approach to the endeavor.[39] The volume is not completely devoted to leisure, however, and includes a section on the kitchen garden as well as some—importantly not all—medicinal uses for the plants. If we keep an eye to Parkinson's conception of a largely female audience in the *Paradisus*, metonymically represented by the queen, against the imagined male audience of the *Theatrum*, we may gain insight into Parkinson's purpose.

[38] In associating the realm of pleasure with Grandmother Eve, Henrietta Maria, and all else female, Parkinson's terrestrial paradise replicates motifs found in literary representations of such quasi-paradisal spaces. Most overtly, Grandmother Eve's focus on herbal "pleasures" is reminiscent of Acrasia and her island in the twelfth canto of Book II of the *Faerie Queene*, in which some version of the word "pleasure" or "pleasant" occurs eighteen times. Spenser's description of the island as the place "where Pleasure dwelles in sensuall delights," and "the most daintie Paradise on ground, / It selfe doth offer to his sober eye, / In which all pleasures plenteously abound" may certainly resonate in reading Parkinson's *Paradisus*. Edmund Spenser, *The Faerie Queene*, ed. Thomas P. Roche, Jr. (London: Penguin, 1978), II.xii.1.8 and II.xii.58.1–3. In such a lineage, Acrasia becomes a type of Eve who is then recovered (and aged) through Parkinson's "Grandmother Eve." What is more, Acrasia's island is strewn with "the ornaments of *Floraes* pride" (171), a pride that may allude to women's vanity, an aspect of plant use dominant in the Garden of Pleasure in the *Paradisus*. But Parkinson is no Guyon. He actually constructs, not destroys, his earthly paradise; even though it concentrates on "pleasures" and "delights," its walls are not as permeable as those of Acrasia's bower.

[39] See Munroe, *Gender and the Garden*.

In the light of his conceived gendered audience, a comparison of Parkinson's two entries—one from the *Paradisus*, the other from the *Theatrum*—on Cyclamen or "Sowebread," for example, can be most illuminating. As the lists of plant uses in the *Paradisus*, because of the book's focus on cultivation, are significantly shorter than those found in the *Theatrum*, one can assume that certain knowledge is being omitted or held back. Within the 1629 discussion of "Sowebread," the list of medicinal/household uses of the flower consists of three sentences, the first being a general summary and the last two being more specifically directed toward women's perceived concerns: "It is vsed also for women in long and hard trauels, where there is danger, to accelerate the birth, either the roote or the leafe being applyed. But for any amorous effects, I hold it meere fabulous" (199). By comparison, the virtues for sowbread as described in Parkinson's second volume take up half a folio page, a list which includes a relation of the help it provides in childbirth but nothing about "amorous effects," interestingly included in the text with fewer entries. Instead *Theatrum* includes a discussion of the ancient authorities Dioscorides, Galen, and Pliny and their belief that sowbread could be used to bring about an abortion (1365). Parkinson controls the knowledge that comes into his terrestrial paradise, determining the kinds of medical procedures practiced there. Whether or not this treatment by Parkinson represents an instance in "agnotology," "the study of cultural ignorance," as Londa Schiebinger has argued in her study of the peacock flower,[40] Parkinson's editorial decisions and his presentation of the content in the separate volumes seem to be indicative of the ways certain kinds of knowledge were suppressed in certain contexts. While it is true that the differences between the texts' foci determine the relative length of the lists of virtues, the decisions made by the author regarding which virtues are carried forward and which are left behind can nonetheless be significant. Having gendered his readership, providing a negative example in Grandmother Eve and a positive one in Henrietta Maria, Parkinson contains certain practices within the enclosed garden while keeping others outside its walls.[41]

In presenting his study of plants in two books, and by differently gendering those volumes, Parkinson propagates two versions of the herbal tradition. One version, the one that preserved knowledge of the delights found in plants, he mainly designates feminine; the other, which focuses on textual debates and medicinal remedies, he describes as "manlike." Herbal histories have replicated this division by keeping the *Paradisus* in a separate category altogether, relegating it to the company of gardening manuals, whereas the *Theatrum* is most often

---

[40] Londa Schiebinger, *Plants and Empire: Colonial Bioprospecting in the Atlantic World* (Cambridge, Massachusetts: Harvard University Press, 2004), 18.

[41] Cf. Schiebinger's reading of Andrew Boorde's 1598 *Breviary of Health* in *Plants and Empire*, 7, n. 35. See also medical historian John M. Riddle, who discusses how texts preserve and control the use of contraceptives and abortifacients in Europe, *Eve's Herbs: A History of Contraception and Abortion in the West* (Cambridge, Massachusetts: Harvard University Press, 1997).

cited as Parkinson's legitimate herbal.[42] The only herbal historian who counters this tendency is one of the first, Eleanour Rohde, but even those who discuss the *Paradisus* "strictly" as a gardening manual admit that much of the book follows a loose herbal format, giving the description, time of bloom, names, and virtues of each plant.[43] Parkinson himself complicates this binary when he presents herbal knowledge as "what Herbes and Fruits were fit, eyther for Meate or Medicine, for Vse or for Delight," gendering "meate" and "delight" as feminine through the figures of Grandmother Eve and the kitchen and "medicine" and "use" as masculine through the figure of Adam, and intertwines the seeming separateness of the tasks in his chiasmic presentation. While most of the plants presented in *Paradisus* reappear in the *Theatrum*, many entries in the *Theatrum* represent the delights and household use meant for the *Paradisus*, albeit as witnessed in ladies or countrywomen versus the more direct use recommended in the "garden of pleasure." Similarly, as Bushnell considers in her study of the *Paradisus*, the early volume conceives of a partly gentleman readership in the way it develops a sense of the professional gardener.[44] Because of this interrelation between the texts, I would suggest that the *Paradisus* is not separate from but is rather central to Parkinson's total herbal project. Relegating delight into female hands through a volume loosely herbal-like, he is able to designate his magnum opus "manlike" and determine the course of herbals—particularly his own—to come. Indeed, at the end of his epistle to the reader in the *Paradisus*, the author promises a "fourth Part" (*Paradisus* containing plants of the pleasure garden, kitchen garden, and orchard) in a future volume, the working title for which is "A Garden of Simples," what becomes the *Theatrum* ("To the Covrteovs Reader," n. p.).

What Parkinson did not count on, however, is the intervention of Thomas Johnson's re-edition of Gerard's *Herball* (1633) in the establishment of the English tradition, an intervention that may have heightened Parkinson's need to assert the "manlike" qualities of his work. "Very much Enlarged and Amended" by Johnson, the 1633 *Herball*, reprinted in 1636, attempts to smooth out the errors made in Gerard's 1597 text, which Gerard rushed to print prematurely. Much has been made (as we will see, virulently in Parkinson's entries in the *Theatrum*) of how little of Gerard's *Herball* is actually Gerard's, depending as it does largely on the translations of Dodoens's Latin text *Stirpium Historiae Pemptades Sex*

---

42 For example, in their surveys of herbals, Arber, *Herbals*, and Anderson, *An Illustrated History of the Herbals*, discuss the *Theatrum Botanicum* exclusively, while Rebecca Bushnell's analysis in *Green Desire* of early modern gardening manuals notes that "at first glance, the book [*Paradisus*] resembles the folio herbals of its time" (59) but, because of her focus, concludes that Parkinson is "a writer recording his thoughts on what it meant to compose a gardening book as opposed to an herbal" (61) and does not consider its relationship to the later *Theatrum*.

43 Rohde, *Old English Herbals*, 142; Bushnell, *Green Desire*, 61.

44 Bushnell, *Green Desire*, 124–26.

(1583) started by Dr. Priest,[45] but many (including Johnson) attempted to promote Gerard's popularity by emphasizing the precedents he sets. Johnson keeps the prefatory materials from the original edition intact, adding only one—though extensive—piece, his address to the reader. In that address, Johnson says, almost as if directly distinguishing his text from Parkinson's *Paradisus* printed four years before, that he "will not speake of the many and various obiects of delight that these [plants] present to the senses."[46] He goes on to describe his intent for his preface, to "acquaint you from what Fountaines this Knowledge may be drawne, by shewing what Authours haue deliuered to vs the Historie of Plants, and after what manner they haue done it" (sig. **2v). What follows is a long list of male herbalists. The list starts with Solomon, touches on the Greek and Roman authorities, explains the cross-germination between continental sources, nods to Turner, Henry Lyte's translation of Rembert Dodoen's *Crŭijdeboeck* and Parkinson, and *ends* with the translation of Dodoens by Dr. Priest, Gerard's edition, and Johnson's own contributions. Johnson acknowledges that he has inserted his edition between Parkinson's two volumes, "refer[ring]" his "Reader addicted to these delights [gardening and preserving]" to the *Paradisus* and adding as a seeming afterthought, "He [Parkinson] also promised another worke, the which I thinke by this time is fit for the Presse" (sig. ***1r). By excluding the discussion of delight from his own preface and confining the *Paradisus*, and thus Parkinson, to that conversation, Johnson undermines Parkinson's future authority by publishing his more authoritative edition of Gerard ahead of Parkinson's second volume.

Even as Parkinson has prepared his reader for the masculinization of his second book in the feminization of his first, the effectual hyper-masculinization of *Theatrum Botanicum* seems to be trying to compensate for Johnson's relegating its author to the garden of delight and beating him—by seven years—to the press and thus to precedence. In the juxtaposition of Parkinson's "an Herbal of a Large Extent" to Johnson's "Very Much Enlarged" version of Gerard and in reading Parkinson's dedication of his "Manlike Worke" to Charles I, one cannot help but feel that Parkinson is overcompensating.[47] *Theatrum*'s architectural frontispiece seems to respond to Parkinson's "manlike" directive: at the same time it is

---

45 Gerard enthusiast Marcus Woodward (*Gerard's Herball: The Essence thereof Distilled by Marcus Woodward* [London: Gerald Howe, 1927]), writes, "Gerard has been harshly judged for failing to acknowledge the source of his Herbal's inspiration; but . . . plagiarism was rife in those days, and we do not find Shakespeare making acknowledgement of the originals of his plays. The Herbal owes its charm to our Author" (xv). For an extended discussion of Gerard's "competitive stance" against herbalists to whom he was indebted, especially Mathias L'Obel, see Harkness, *The Jewel House*, 52.

46 Thomas Johnson, "To the reader," in John Gerard, *The Herball or Generall Historie of Plantes* (1633), sig. **2v. Subsequent references included in the text. Anna Parkinson's biography of John Parkinson, *Nature's Alchemist: John Parkinson, Herbalist to Charles I* (London: Frances Lincoln Limited, 2007), touches on this rivalry with Johnson (231–42).

47 Parkinson, *Theatrum Botanicum*, second title page.

reminiscent of the 1633 Gerard (and a line of herbals before them), it is intensely constrained in comparison with the much more fluid lines of the *Paradisus* (Figure 1.2).[48] Even though at the end of the *Paradisus* he had submitted a much more attractive—if more feminine—title, *The Garden of Simples*, for his second volume, Parkinson chooses *Theatrum Botanicum*, which as Rohde notes, "sounds hard and chilling" and in early seventeenth-century England has associations with male-only performance. The substantially calved figures of Adam and Solomon are four times the size of the allegorical female figures representing the four continents in each corner.[49] The 1633 edition of Gerard has comparable figures of Theophrastus and Dioscorides, who are only double the size of the corresponding Ceres and Pomona above them. While *Paradisus* had its feminine contours, *Theatrum* draws attention to its masculine attributes, of which the author and printer have insured there are many.

Further evidence that the hyper-masculinization of Parkinson's second volume may be related to his rivalry with Gerard is found in the language of patrilineage in his preface. Reminiscent of Turner, Parkinson discusses how he looks to "avoyd and amend" the "many slips and errors crept" into his "Profession" (i.e., apothecary) and describes how those mistakes have passed from generation to generation because "some delight to be obstinate, and because they were bred up in errors, they will not be wiser then their Fathers, but together live and dye in them, yea and condemne that light that others have, because they thinke their darkenesse better" ("To the Reader," n. p.). The use of "delight" hints that something may be going on with Johnson's edition of Gerard here, and stronger proof occurs within the volume itself. For example, in the entry on "The Excressences of the Holme Okes," Parkinson writes that "a third errour rose from *Dodoneus*, that mistooke *Sericam*, and made it *Seta*, whose errour Doctor *Priest*, that translated him into *English* did follow, and gave occasion to *Gerard* so to publish it so in his Herball, in that *Gerard* received that translation from Mr. *Norton* to finish" (1397). Importantly, though Parkinson lists four other "errors" in the historical use of this plant, he names only one other herbalist, "Mesues the Arabian."[50] Parkinson's entry shows Gerard (and following him, Johnson) to be the very sort of "obstinate" herbalist who is "no wiser" than his many fathers and exposes him as a publisher of errors as well as

---

48 For an example of an herbal with similar outlines, see John Prest, *Garden of Eden: The Botanic Garden and the Recreation of Paradise* (New Haven, Connecticut: Yale University Press, 1981), 58. See also Julie Stone Peters, *Theatre of the Book, 1480–1880: Print, Text, and Performance in Europe* (Oxford: Oxford University Press, 2000), for a discussion of "title pages whose organizing trope was the architectural portico ringed by animated figures" (106).

49 Rohde, *Old English Herbals*, 151–52.

50 See Anderson's discussion of Mesue the Yonger and Serapion the younger, "two famous Arabic authors who are not Arabs at all," *An Illustrated History of Herbals*, 36. What is more, Parkinson does not mention that Johnson amends Gerard's 1597 "bristle" (1160G) to his 1633 "silke" (1343G).

someone, in the words of Turner, "mak[ing] frendes with other mennis trauayles" (sig. *3r). In doing so, it practically bleeds resentment. Thus the language of faulty fathers contributes to the overall gendering of legitimate herbal knowledge, i.e., the *Theatrum*, as male. In this hyper-masculinization, he erodes all things female, arguably to his detriment.[51] Whereas Johnson's edition of Gerard's *Herball* had a second run in 1636 and the *Paradisus* was printed again in 1635 and 1656, *Theatrum Botanicum* was never reprinted in the seventeenth century.

Parkinson reveals his real resentment, however, later in the preface, when he, like Turner before him, articulates a contentious defense against his would-be critics, figured as Momus, who also appears in the last pages of the *Paradisus*:

> One bout more with *Momus* in a Bookesellers shop, for more roome I must not overslip, that would teare this Worke in peeces because I have not followed *Gerards* method, in setting Letters to the severall vertues of the Plants. . . . [T]he bulke of the Booke which if that course had been followed, would have enlarged it well neere halfe as much more; and made it the more unweldy, and likewise the dearer and never a whit better. ("To the Reader," n.p.)

The "method" Parkinson refers to here is Gerard's system of indexing, which helps the reader negotiate a long block of text and seemingly garners Gerard some popularity. Parkinson's defense is logical, but it is also filled with an undeniable, well, anxiety. His work, as an artificial representation of himself, is in danger, Actaeon-like, of being "ripped to pieces" and consequently forgotten. In his defensive stance, he points out that his text is already larger than Gerard's "very much enlarged" herbal, even without "Gerards method."

Because Gerard could be having the final word in the English herbal tradition, it would seem that Parkinson wants to establish a new patrilineage of herbalism, one that begins with himself. In a very literary move, the author tells his book:

> Goe forth now therefore thou issue artificiall of mine, and supply the defect of a Naturall, to beare up thy Fathers name and memory to succeeding ages, and what in thee lyeth effect more good to thy Prince and Country then numerous of others, which often prove rather plagues then profits thereto . . . . ("To the Reader;" n. p.)

That "numerous" other herbals have been published in England speaks to Parkinson's sense of his own belatedness. He thus names them "plagues" to replace them with his remedies and becomes the true "Father" of the English herbal.

---

[51] Rohde asserts that "Parkinson originally intended to entitle it 'A Garden of Simples' and, had he done so, it is at least possible that this work, to which he devoted the greater part of his life, would have achieved the popularity it deserved. . . . In fact, this herbal of Parkinson's is an outstanding proof that a good book may be ruined by a bad title" (*Old English Herbals*, 151).

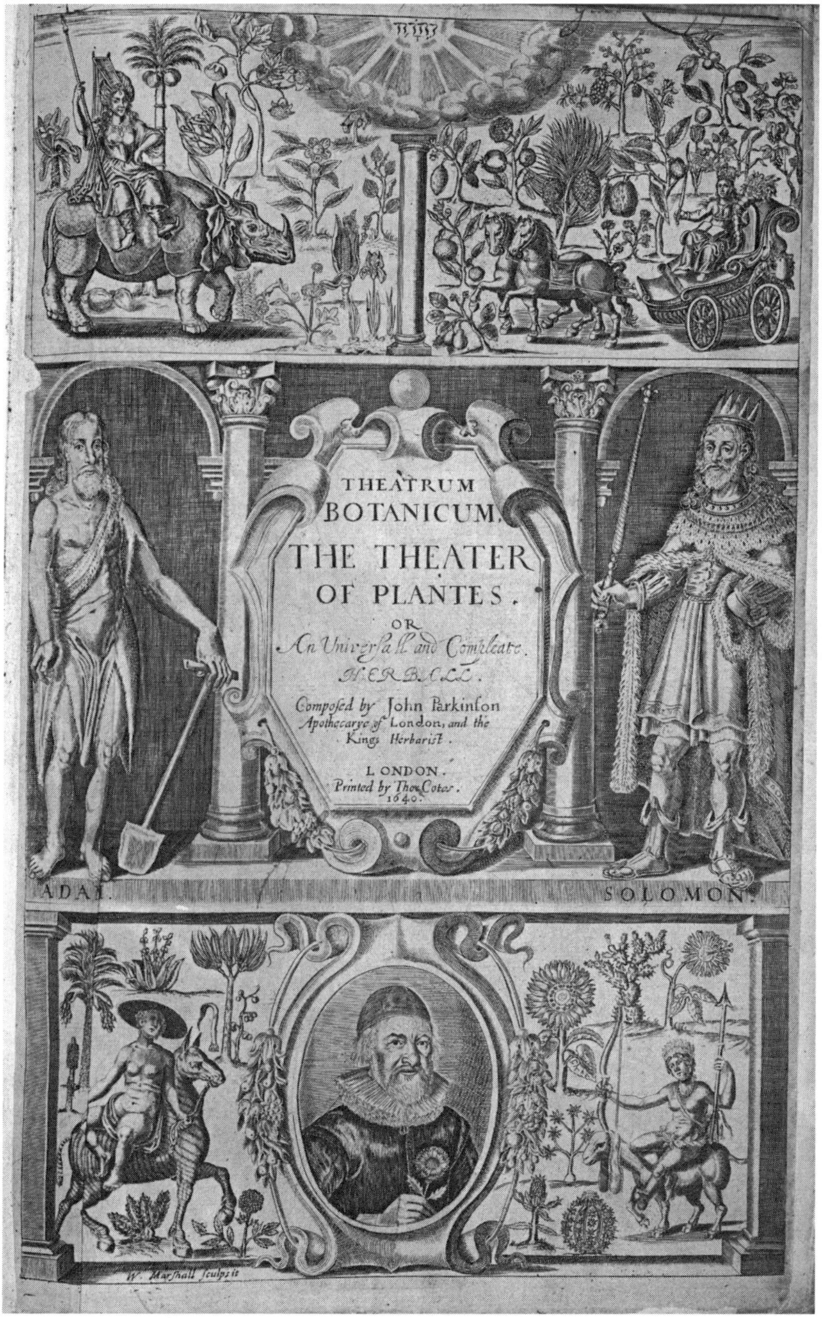

Fig. 1.2 Frontispiece from John Parkinson's *Theatrum Botanicum, the Theater of Plantes* (1640). Courtesy of the Library of Congress.

If this analysis has begun to sound like that of literary rivalry and lineage—particularly in its homosocial aspects—discussed so often by so many, it is unavoidable.[52] While at first it may seem that the gendering of herbal practice has to do with competition between practitioners of different genders, upon closer examination, issues of gender seem to arise in these volumes because of rivalries between authors of the same gender. It follows that if the herbwife in Turner's earlier entry in the English herbal tradition reflects insecurities about the establishment of that tradition relative to continental sources, Parkinson's concerted gendering of his mid-seventeenth-century herbals would come to register tensions internal to the English textual tradition. Because women before 1640 were not part of the English print herbal tradition, they could not intercede in such projections, and as a result print authority was defeminized at the same time as it became masculinized. It is important to note, however, that while it is seductive to impose a narrative about the subjugation of women on such gendering of the text, the language in the text has much more to do with dramas played out within the textual tradition itself than with any censure by the College of Physicians or any witch trial. That is, in establishing the tradition, these authors may inadvertently contribute to the discourse that excludes women from the practice of institutionalized medicine, but their rhetorical motives are more immediate and are clearly textually derived. Even though some may deem this rhetoric as more insidious than the more overt exclusionary practices, my purpose in exposing the rhetoric as rhetoric is to weaken its "truth-telling" claims by revealing the insecurities underneath.[53] Understanding how and to what ends the female practitioner comes to be represented in establishing the tradition is essential for understanding that tradition.

As the tradition develops its conventions, it also establishes its readership. We have seen figures for the female reader–practitioner in Queen Henrietta Maria and, at the outset of this chapter, Anne Wilbraham. Against these literate women are foiled the illiterate practitioners represented in the text, the "old wife," the grandmother, the "cousener," and the witch, all depicted as threats in the text yet all unable to read it. In the next two sections, we see how the tradition further defines its Christian gentlewoman reader through counterposition to the pagan and uneducated witch and through alignment with the educated and charitable queen. In thus creating a position for the gentlewoman practitioner, however limited, the herbal tradition further exposes its anxieties about the establishment of textual authority in a medical environment that is as fluid as it is ungeneralizable.

---

52 See, for example, James S. Shapiro's *Rival Playwrights: Marlowe, Jonson, Shakespeare* (New York: Columbia University Press, 1991) and Raphael Falco's analysis of literary lineage in *Conceived Presences: Literary Genealogy in Renaissance England* (Amherst: University of Massachusetts Press, 1991). For a discussion of the homosocial in literary relations see Eve Kosofsky Sedgwick, *Between Men: English Literature and Male Homosocial Desire* (New York: Columbia University Press, 1985).

53 Shapin, *Social History of Truth*. See also Bushnell, *Green Desire*.

Circe and Malevolent Herbal Practice

In the establishment of the print tradition of the English herbal, we have thus far seen how figures of female practical authority in herbal medicine can be introduced in order to take on the textual fallibility that accompanies translation and transmission. It now should be conceivable that other representations of female practitioners found in the herbals reveal less about female medical practice and more about insecurities surrounding the printing of the herbal text. In this section, we will consider how representations of the witch in the herbal tradition expose anxieties about the ways in which the herbal text may contribute to unregulated—and dangerous—herbal practice. We have considered how in Parkinson's project, sensual and amateur applications of plants come to be identified with women's herbal use. A different but related treatment of female owners of herbal knowledge depends on culturally repeated structures of dominance found in the ancient myth of Circe, Mercury, and Ulysses.[54] An examination of how this mythic structure enters the vernacular herbal uncovers the intersection between the discussion of witchcraft in the early modern period and the establishment of the English print herbal tradition.

Once again, we begin with the work of William Turner, this time turning to his dedicatory epistle to the Duke of Somerset from his 1551 *A New Herball*. In that epistle, Turner invokes the herbwife in a way that anticipates but differs from his reference to her in 1568. As in the lost-horse passage, Turner responds to his imagined critics. Distinctive from the lost-horse passage, however, is the way the "old wyfe" here exists as both gatherer and keeper—but not distributor—of herbal knowledge:

> Other[s] will thinke it vnwysely done. . . .[B]y occasyon of thys boke euery man, nay euery old wyfe will presume, not without the mordre of many, to practyse Phisick. To whom I make thys answer, by a questyon, how many surgianes and apothecaries are there in England, which can vnderstande Plini in latin . . . of the names descriptions and natures of herbes? And when as they haue no latin to come by the knowledge of herbes: whether all the Phisicians of England (sauyng very few) committ not y[e] knowledge of herbes vnto the potecaries or no, as the potecaries do to the olde wyues, that gather herbes, & to the grossers, whylse they send all their receytes vnto the potecary, not beyng present their to se, whether the potecary putteth all that shuld be in to the receyt or no? Then when as if the potecari for lack of knowledge of the latin tong, is ignorant in herbes: and putteth . . . many a good mā by ignorance in ieopardy of his life . . .? [W]hen as by hauyng an herball in English all these euelles myght be auoyded: whether were it better, that many men shuld be killed, or the herbal shuld be set out in

[54] My discussion here is related to but different from William Kerwin's discussion of "Medea's traces" in *Beyond the Body: The Boundaries of Medicine and English Renaissance Drama* (Amherst: University of Massachusetts Press, 2005), 62–96.

> Englysh. . . . Dioscorides wrote hys great herball in greke . . . Dyd Dioscorides . . . gyye occasiō for euery old wyfe to take in hād the practise of Phisick? Dyd [he] gyue any iust occasyon of murther? . . . If [he] gaue no occasyon vnto euery old wyfe to practyse physike, then gyue I none. . . . (sig. A3r–A3v)[55]

This passage taps into a larger top-down cultural anxiety about unregulated (often female) participation in herbal medicine. Through his defensive stance, Turner is able to articulate his ultimate goal, which is to divorce those belonging to legitimate medical institutions from their dependence on faulty knowledge. He depicts a cultural practice in which herbal knowledge is shared orally and is thus not controllable. In saying that Dioscorides did not give occasion "for euery old wyfe to take in ha[n]d the practise of Phisick," he does not imply that women did not practice medicine; he is simply pointing out that their practice had not been dependent on texts. As we have seen in the 1568 preface, the herbal text is meant to *supplant*—not facilitate—the knowledge of the "olde herbe wives," and with the displacement of these old wives will come the domination over all oral preservation of herbal knowledge. It is also important to point out here that the "old wyfe" who would practice physic is not necessarily part of the group of "old wyues, that gather herbes." What these women do have in common is that they both look to make money from the knowledge of herbs; an "old wife" in the period was someone "engaged in the sale of some commodity."[56] That she is also someone of "humble rank" is a point that has increasing importance in this study as the herbal establishes a professional and gentle readership meant to exclude the practitioner of small economic means.

To what extent Turner's displacement and disparagement of the "old wyfe" is meant to allay cultural anxieties about orally propagated knowledge and unregulated practice in general can best be explored through the mythic structures of dominance found elsewhere in the herbal texts. These mythic structures reveal how the patriarchal constructions often imbedded in early feminist readings are mythic in their dissemination and have a spectral relationship with actual practice. Given the repeated references to source in the herbal text, it should come as no surprise that classical myth, in this instance that of Odysseus/Ulysses and Circe,

---

55 Wear, *Knowledge and Practice in English Medicine*, concludes about this passage, "Despite Turner relying on local knowledge when compiling his herbals, there was no sense of the 'olde wyves' informing the apothecaries and physicians. Instead, Turner envisaged only a top-down dissemination of information," 62. On the contrary, Turner "envisaged" the bottom-up "dissemination" in his later work when his rhetorical strategies were differently directed. That Turner presents both as "truths" begs the question of what really is being represented. Wendy Wall also discusses this passage in *Staging Domesticity: Household Work and English Identity in Early Modern Drama* (Cambridge: Cambridge University Press, 2002), 33.

56 "wife, n[1a]" *The Oxford English Dictionary*, 2nd ed. 1989, *OED Online*, Oxford University Press, http://dictionary.oed.com/cgi/entry/50285384 (accessed March 2, 2009).

comes to inform the self-perception of educated male medical authority, especially with regard to its illiterate female counterparts.

In Homer's epic, Odysseus' men explore the island of Aeaea to find Circe singing and weaving in her bower. She invites them in, slips a drug into their wine, taps them with her wand, and turns them into pigs. One man, Eurylochus, does not drink the wine and escapes to tell Odysseus. Odysseus sets out to confront the witch. On the hero's way to this confrontation, the messenger god Hermes intercepts him and gives Odysseus an herb (in Homer, it is called "moly") to protect him against the herbal potions of Circe. Through this herb, Odysseus is able to deflect Circe's spell and consequently overcome her. In doing so, Odysseus gains Circe's help in spells and soothsaying for the rest of his voyage. In this myth, we find the structures of dominance and appropriation that underpin the herbal project. Malevolent, unregulated female herbal authority is subjugated to divinely sanctioned male herbal authority, which then goes on to acquire knowledge from that female authority. These structures appear both overtly and covertly throughout the herbal texts as a kind of justification for the dissemination of textual herbal knowledge. In that dissemination, the Hermes-like herbalist gives his reader a kind of preservative against illegitimate female practice.

Through the lens of the Circe–Hermes–Odysseus myth, the 1568 passage from Turner quoted in the previous section takes on new dimensions. In one sense, the herbwife is the witch from whom Hermes/the herbalist grants protection. That the "olde herbe wives" already have a hand in medical practice and do not refer to any book to do so (neither does Circe) is one of the central tensions in the herbal text. Both the 1551 and 1568 passages express the anxiety that herbal knowledge in the hands of women is a bad thing against which men need protection, and in providing the structure through which that malevolent force can be contained, the myth provides a means through which this anxiety may be addressed. In the 1568 passage, Turner looks to remove the herbwife from the hierarchy of herbal knowledge altogether. In essence, Turner's proposal is to take the place of Hermes, give the apothecary the moly-like herbal, and make the Circe–herbwife powerless and irrelevant (part of her power has already been taken away in making her old). In thus re-articulating the hierarchy of herbalism from Physician–Apothecary–Herbwife to Herbalist–Physician/Apothecary as we have seen above, he does away with the malevolent-because-unregulated force that cannot be trusted.

In the interest of assertions about status, the early modern herbal often presents the illiterate practical authority's disempowerment at the hands of classical textual authority, a dynamic that is problematized by the presence of non-textual authority within and around those classical texts. A closer examination of the manipulation of the mythic structures will help us to see how the problematic coexistence of female/oral and male/written authorities persists within the English herbal at the same time that these binaries break down and the structures alter.

In the herbals, the myth of Circe is most overtly present in its retellings by Apuleius Barbarus (fourth or fifth century C. E.?) and Pliny (first century C. E.) as represented in entries for mullein and moly, respectively.[57] The 1578 translation of Rembert Dodoens by Henry Lyte, *A Nievve Herball, or Historie of Plantes*, most faithfully relates the passage from Apuleius: "Mercury gaue Mulleyn to Vlysses, whan he came neare to the inchanteresse Circe, to the ende that by the vertue of Mulleyn he might be preserued against all the enchantments or witchings of Circe."[58] Then under "moly," *A Nievve Herball* relates to the reader that "Moly is also excellent against enchauntementes, as Plinie . . . do[es] testifie, saying, That Mercurie reuealed or shewed it to Ulysses, whereby he escaped all the enchauntments of Circe, the Magicien" (509b). In these overt references to the myth, classical myth metonymically represents the more extensive body of texts from which the early modern herbalist derives his authority. In less open ways, moreover, the herbals can also mirror the structures of the myth. For example, Lyte's/Dodoens's entries "Alysson" (108c) and "Rhamnus" (696c) make a claim for the power of those herbs against witchcraft, but unlike with moly and mullein, these entries do not give a named source, coming only from "some" who "hold" this to be true. Thus Dodoens's text works to counteract the malevolent, female use of herbs in two ways. First, the classically authorized entries present us with an image of legitimate (Mercury-sanctioned *and* textually verified) use of medicine by men (Ulysses and the Physician) overcoming the malevolent and female uses of herbs by women (Circe and illiterate practitioners). Secondly, the textualization of oral or anonymous traditions subverts the powers of the tradition it is codifying; that is, in relating how the reader can protect him/herself from witches, from illiterate old women (as represented in the period) who manipulate herbs, these texts counteract the potency of those witches' herbal knowledge. The witch is disempowered by the textual dissemination of knowledge against her. Implicit in this logic, however, is that she has the power to begin with, powers that precede the text and reside outside it.

It should come as no surprise that these moments intersect with the larger discussion of witchcraft in the period, a discussion that also argues against unregulated (illiterate) practice of herbal medicine while championing the legitimate (learned) practices of physicians. The following passage from George Gifford's *A Discourse of the subtill Practises of Deuilles by VVitches and Sorcerers* (1587) encapsulates the cultural tension between regulated and unregulated medical practitioners that also informs the debate on witchcraft.[59] Notice in particular how Gifford elides the difference between cunning woman, wise woman, and witch:

---

[57] See Jerry Stannard, "The Plant Called Moly,"*Herbs and Herbalism in the Middle Ages and Renaissance*, ed. Katherine E. Stannard and Richard Kay (Aldershot, Hampshire: Ashgate Variorum, 1999), 254–307, for a discussion of the debate over moly's identification.

[58] Dodoens, *A Nievve Herball*, 121.

[59] Pelling, *Medical Conflicts*.

> I will … lay open the filthie vices which the people are drawne into by witchcraft …. A man is sicke, his sicknesse doth linger vpon him. Some doe put into his head that he is bewitched. He is counselled to send vnto a cunning woman. She saith he is forspoken indéede, she prescribeth them what to vse, there must be some charme and sorcerie vsed. The partie findeth ease, & is a glad man, he taketh it that he hath made a good market, it was a luckie hower whē he sent to that woman. … The wise woman with her familer was too strong for him. O that the hearts of men were not turned into the hearts of beasts, but that they would consider.[60]

Gifford criticizes this "vice" through the logic of the Circe, Ulysses, and Mercury myth. Most overtly, he does so through the exclamation "O that the hearts of men were not turned into the hearts of beasts," connecting the wisewomen's practice with Circe's metamorphosis of Ulysses's men into swine. As the passage continues, Gifford anticipates his critics, but unlike Turner's, his critics argue *for* the lay practice of medicine by women. One can imagine that these critics are not doctors of any shade; they rather come from the camp of the patient who cannot afford access to the costly physician:

> Some man will replye that this is a commō thing and well tried by experience, that many in great distresse haue bin reléeued and recouered by sending vnto such wise men or wise women, when they could not tel what should els become of them …. Shall not men take helpe where they can find it? Why do men go vnto Phisicions? Let it be graunted that men finde helpe by Witches. Yet this must néedes be graūted, that as it is for the most part a plague and token of Gods displeasure, where he hath power graunted him to vexe: so is it a more heauie iudgement, which the wicked world hath deserued, that he is suffered to heale. For now they cannot say that the Lord is their health and saluation, but their Phisicion is the deuill…. O miserable health so recouered. … He which seeketh helpe in sicknes at the hands of a Phisicion, doth that which is lawfull being ordeyned of God. For he hath giuen the nature & properties vnto things, which shall serue for medicine.[61]

Gifford also invokes the myth through calling those who seek legitimate practices as doing that which is "lawfull being ordeyned of God." The pagan deity bearing the protective moly or mullein has been replaced by the Christian God, who "hath giuen the nature & properties vnto things, which shall serve for medicine" (recalling for us Parkinson's allusion to Genesis in the *Paradisus*). The difference here is an important one. What protects the individual is not an herb; it is the trust in God-ordained, physician-administered medicine rather than in the wily workings

---

60 George Gifford, *A Discourse of the subtill Practises of Devilles by VVitches and Sorcerers* (London, 1587), sigs. H1r–H1v.

61 Gifford, *A Discourse of the subtill Practises of Devilles*, sig. H1v.

of the Circean wisewoman. As we shall see, this difference is significant in the development of the herbal texts' simultaneous incorporation of and domination over lay practical knowledge.

The intersection between the witchcraft pamphlets and the early stages of the English vernacular herbal depicts a world in which the common man may be subjected to the malevolent/ignorant and female use of herbs and consequently emasculated. In the works of Gifford, Turner, and Lyte/Dodoens, the male-authored text intervenes and protects the victim through learned medicine. The writer of the witchcraft pamphlet introduces the figure of the physician as holder of that knowledge; the herbalist presents the authoritative herbal itself. In both cases the text and the knowledge it brings provide the ultimate protection.[62]

In the later herbals of Gerard and Parkinson, a Christian God begins to transform pagan mythic structures. In the example from Gifford, those who submit to the wisewoman's wiles become part of the mythic structure, become animal-like or in need of protection, but those who turn to God-sanctioned remedies from the outset escape it. Similarly, the Circe–Ulysses pattern begins to shift in the later herbals. Coming from a shared source in Dodoens,[63] a variation on Lyte's mullein entry exists in Gerard's 1597 *Herball*, and the differences between the Lyte and Gerard translations of Apuleius complicate this analysis thus far. Instead of describing the transmission of herbal knowledge from Mercury to Ulysses, Gerard writes "*Apuleius* reporteth a tale of *Vlysses*, *Mercurie*, and the inchauntresse *Circe*, and their vse of these herbes in their incantations and witchcrafts" (632). Gerard places an egalitarian witchcraft in the hands of all three figures, thus distancing himself from pagan practice. This reworking of Apuleius does not undo the gendered dynamics discussed above, however. On the contrary, Gerard's later version is a development, if not an enactment, of Lyte's earlier rendition, one that replaces the pagan deities and practices with male Christian purpose and medicine. Admittedly, the difference between Lyte and Gerard is subtle. While Lyte's version presents the subjugation of witchcraft in the terms of witchcraft, making the reader a more potent Ulysses in the face of encountered malevolence, Gerard's text denies the existence of malevolent power in the first place, and in so doing, weakens the pagan tradition behind it. In rhetorical moves similar to the witchcraft pamphlets, the later herbalists show how, in the Christian colonial era, Greek tradition is represented as Circean in its superstitions.

---

[62] Indeed, while the herbal lists plants that act as protection against witchcraft, many of the pamphlets from the witchcraft debates end with a supposed "cure for" or "preservative against" witchcraft, often having to do with religious practice and stalwart faith. For examples, see Gifford, *Discourse*, sig. J2v; William Perkins, *A Discourse of the Damned Art of Witchcraft* (Cambridge, 1608), 174; Henry Holland, *A Treatise Against VVitchcraft* (Cambridge, 1590), sig. H1r.

[63] More interesting still, there is no reference to Apuleius in Dodoens's Latin text, *Stirpivm Historiae Pemptades Sex* (Antwerp, 1583), which is purportedly Gerard's source.

In this way, the figure of the witch, often but not always gendered female, comes to take on all of the superstitions inherited through the ancient/continental herbal traditions. This dynamic is similar to the ways in which the ignorant herbwife comes to take on the errors of the continental sources and is made clearer through a quick juxtaposition of Gerard's entries on mugwort and vervain. On mugwort, the author adds commentary to his source in Dodoens's *Pemptades Sex*, which simply relates the passage from Pliny about its semi-magical powers to give energy to the weary: "Many other fantasticall deuices inuented by Poets are to be seene in the workes of auncient writers, tending to Witchcraft and sorcerie, and the great dishonor of God, wherefore I do of purpose omit them as things vnworthie of my recording or your reuiewing" (946D). Similarly, Gerard's entry on vervain or verbena refers to the practice of the folkloric wisewoman, "mother Bumbie," who is superstitiously exacting in the number of knots and sprigs used in fighting fever, and comments, "Many odde olde wiues fables are written of Veruaine tending to witchcraft and sorcerie, which you may reade else where, for I am not willing to trouble your eares with reporting such trifles, as honest eares abhorre to heare" (581C). Gerard thus frames his propensity to resist any inclination toward "witchcraft and sorcerie" as a progressive and godly practice, again placing the beliefs of the wisewoman and witch within the categories of deceit, triviality, and sin.

At this point I would like to address two aspects of mythmaking important for this argument: namely, the purported historical realities of the witch as healer and the witch as primarily female. While Diane Purkiss has caused us to rethink the feminist stereotype that has occurred through invested interpretation, my interest here is not so much in reasserting the stereotype but rather in uncovering how the stereotype is embedded in mythic structures in the period.[64] Circe's herbal prowess becomes a prototype for malevolent female herbal practice in general—in the Ovidian version of the myth, she is even first seen sorting herbs. The Circean prototype then informs discussions in the period of the cunning woman who incorporated herbs into her healing practice. In short, we could argue that in the debates over witchcraft, the cunning woman or wisewoman is made synonymous with the witch, thus making a certain class of women's herbal practice, that by the unlearned, Circean in its aspect. Alternatively, we could argue that the Circean precedent informs the debates over witchcraft, thus affecting the interpretation of the wisewoman's herbal practice as witchlike.

Secondly, although scholars such as Lara Apps and Andrew Gow have justifiably questioned the readiness with which early modern scholars identify the witch as female, in certain circumstances this gendering has mythic precedents that are then invoked for pointedly rhetorical effects.[65] For example, even though

---

64 Diane Purkiss, *The Witch in History: Early Modern and Twentieth-Century Representations* (New York: Routledge, 1996), 7–8.

65 Lara Apps and Andrew Gow, *Male Witches in Early Modern Europe* (Manchester: Manchester University Press, 2003).

Gifford follows his image of the wisewoman healing through herbs and charms with another of a cunning man who finds a lost object, he significantly makes the one cunning person giving medicine female and ties her to the myth of Circe ("the hearts of men . . . into the hearts of beasts"). Thus the discussion of witchcraft becomes intertwined with herbal practice as the witch/Circe becomes a kind of female herbal authority.

By the time his texts were published, Parkinson, as Eleanour Rohde reports, "regards the use of herbs against witchcraft as sheer foolishness."[66] Parkinson's disparagement of popular belief, however, does not mean that he is able entirely to exclude those beliefs. He may count the discussion of witchcraft as "foolishness," "but," Rohde continues, "he is the only herbalist who gives us a potion which 'resisteth such charmes or the like witchery, that is used in such drinkes that are given to produce love.'"[67] Parkinson tellingly places any continued witchery in the arena of love and "delight." Circe has returned, but she is no longer the practitioner who threatens to undermine the growing medical establishment; she is the exotic bearer of love potions and, perhaps, something a little more dangerous and ultimately foreign. Excluded from Rohde's discussion of witchcraft protection is the name of the plant in question, and the specific nature of this anti-charm, called "Indian Spanish Counterpoyson" (*Theatrum* 421), points to the final stage in the witch's transforming role in the English herbal tradition. Parkinson translates its virtues and awkward name from the Nicolás Monardes's work on "New World" plants, and the anti-charm potentials were purportedly related to the Spaniard by the natives of Peru, a transmission expressed in the original entry through the simple parenthetical "they say" (422).

Further evidence that Parkinson expands the witch's role in the tradition to include not only pagan beliefs of ancients but also the sometimes dangerous practices of other cultures can be found in the *Paradisus*. Under the virtues of "thorn apple" in the *Theatrum*, Parkinson emphasizes its powers in dissolving kidney or gallstones; as another indicator of the differences between the volumes, in the "Garden of pleasant Flowers" of the *Paradisus*, under the same plant he relates the following:

> The East Indian lasciuious women performe strange acts with the seed . . . giuing it their husbands to drinke. The whole plant, but especially the seed, is of a very cold and soporiferous quality, procuring sleep and distraction of senses. A few of the seeds steeped and giuen in drinke, will cause them that take it to seem starke drunke or dead drunke, which fit will within a few hours weare away, and they recouer their senses again, as a drunken man raysed after sleep from his wine. It may therefore (in my opinion) be of safe and good vse to one; that is to haue

---

66 Rohde, *Old English Herbals*, 155.

67 Rohde, *Old English Herbals*, 155. The original quote is from Parkinson, *Theatrum Botanicum*, 422, though it reads "procure love."

> a legge or an arme cut off . . . otherwise I hold it not fit to be vsed without great caution. (362)

What these "strange acts" are exactly is difficult to tell, but the description of the East Indian women as "lasciuious" seems to imply that it has to do with the infidelity of the wife as her husband is distracted or asleep. Supporting this claim is Parkinson's suggested usage of this soporific effect "to haue a legge or an arme cut off," a kind of displaced castration of the patient-cuckold. The idea that her sexual potency and his virtual castration bear some relation to the "barbaric" Circe and the unmanning of Ulysses' men as they are turned into pigs is borne out in the conclusion of the entry, which relates that thorn-apple also may be used "to take away any hot inflammations, being made vp into a salue or ointment with … Hogs larde" (362). Again, women's use of these texts could be dangerous, which explains the directive for thorn apple not "to be used without great caution." Thus Parkinson interposes himself and his god-like authority against the malevolent use of herbs through the text. He becomes a kind of Mercury to the Ulysses-like reader, or in the case of the female readership courted by the *Paradisus*, directs the would-be Circe away from subversive practice. The author's words of caution, however, do not entirely counteract the potentials created through the story: that in the wrong hands, the seeds of thorn-apple may cause "distraction[s]."

The female practitioner as considered thus far in this chapter—herbwife, witch, or East Indian woman—represents certain displaced anxieties about herbal publication. Beyond the actual depiction of the exotic other as witch, the Eastern woman here could be seen to represent the subversive, uncontrollable powers of herbs themselves, which could make men into beasts and which became more mystified with the expansion of herbal knowledge through colonization, as seen particularly in Parkinson's *Theatrum* but also as early as Gerard. For evidence that these powers are associated with the exotic other, one need think only of the extensive debates on tobacco, in which one pamphleteer derides the way "intoxicating *Tobacco fumes* are able (in an vnperceivable and Circean manner) to transforme nobilitie into gentrie, gentrie into yeomanrie."[68]

With tobacco we return to the entry from Elizabeth Digby's recipe book discussed in the introduction and Gerard's directive against witches and "charmers." Unlike Parkinson, who later confines female usage, Gerard gives "women of all sorts"—i.e., those who can read—privileged access to perceivably dangerous drugs. The witches who hold knowledge of herbs represent not simply competition in the eyes of the herbalist and physician; they also come to represent the thing more feared, the uncontrollable dimension of self-administration and unregulated practice that these texts could facilitate. This insight is related to that achieved by Edith Snook,

[68] John Deacon, *Tobacco Tortvred, or, the Filthie Fvme of Tobacco Refined* (London, 1616), 66, quoted by Kristen Brookes in "Inhaling the Alien: Race and Tobacco in Early Modern England" (paper delivered at SAMLA conference, Roanoke, Virginia, November 13, 2004).

who, in responding to Mary Ellen Lamb, writes that "representation of female reading is . . . the manifestation of a wide range of concerns around literacy—about vernacularity, religion, class, and nationalism—so that, sometimes, female sexuality is also a trope through which to speak about other sources of disquiet."[69] In the context of herbal reading, herbal *practice* is an extension of that reading; thus the female practitioners represented by the authors in part "manifest" the authors' "concerns" about the public nature of their projects. In displacing the anxiety about uncontrolled substance use onto the figure of the old wife, the East Indian woman, and the witch (none of which, importantly, is English-literate), the herbalist creates a figure that is controllable, distant, hangable. Godlike, the herbalists attempt to control self-administration by the herbal properties they do and do not represent and by the illegitimate—often female—practitioners they censure.

So far, in examining the position of female herbal authority within male-authored herbal texts, we have come to see how female herbal usage—particularly that of uneducated, non-gentry women—is often represented as herbal abuse, that is, as ignorantly filled with errors, lasciviously focused on pleasure, or malevolently meant to cause harm. How much this may reflect actual female herbal practice is nearly impossible to determine. We can see, however, how these negative representations of independent female practice placed on the poor and foreign serve rhetorically to buttress the positive textual version of the gentlewoman practitioner, whose knowledge is textually based and whose practice is charitable and thus circumscribed. As a result, we may be tempted to interpret the female-authored writings in the following chapters as falling into this binary opposition between practice that is economically motivated and thus construed as malevolent, and that which is charitable and thus by association beneficent. Before we see these writings as either capitulating or resistant, however, we must first examine how the seemingly positive models represented in the herbals are no less infused by authorial insecurities than the negative ones.

The Queen and "Dainty" Herbal Practice

Whereas the herbwife and the witch discussed in the previous sections play large roles in Chapter 4, where commerce is seen to affect writing practice, in Chapters 2 and 3, as in this section, the gentlewoman practitioner, who practiced among the poor, her family, and the extended household, is the main focus of analysis. Here the figure of the queen, as metonym for the group of elite female practitioners, takes on the cloaks of charity, maternity, and luxury. Again, however, we should not be shocked if issues of female herbal use become enmeshed with other tensions

---

[69] Edith Snook, *Women, Reading, and the Cultural Politics of Early Modern England* (Aldershot, Hampshire: Ashgate Publishing, 2005), 12.

and anxieties surrounding herbal publication and the domestic is not a simple and apolitical sphere.

Recent studies by Lena Cowen Orlin, Wendy Wall, and Katharine Gillespie have pointed out the cultural potential within the English word "domestic" in the period.[70] Orlin uncovers how the articulation of architectural domestic spaces in the early modern period contributes to the formation of the public (and consequently the private) self. The simultaneous emergence of a sense of national identity and the articulation of housewifely duties in print constitutes the center of Wall's analysis of household manuals and early modern drama. Gillespie's focus on the emergence of liberal philosophy from women's dissent writings in the seventeenth century leads to an instructive discussion of "the ethos of care" within this genre and the role the language of domesticity can play in the articulation of specific religious arguments.[71] The dual sense of the "domestic" as that belonging within a country's boundaries and that within the walls of the household informs the English herbal tradition as well.

In order to explore the multi-dimensionality of gentlewomen's practice as represented in the English vernacular herbals we have examined thus far, this section considers the recurrent appearance of queens or queen-like figures in them. Three of our herbals—those of Turner, Lyte/Dodoens, and Gerard—were published during the reign of Elizabeth I. While this fact certainly accounts in part for the presence of the queen in these herbals, the variation in treatment between and within these volumes signals developments in the textual herbal tradition as it is being established and the relationship between that tradition and developing notions of the domestic in both meanings of that word. Then, not surprisingly, seventeenth-century Parkinson's manipulation of these figures indicates a different moment within the English tradition, one informed by rising political tensions and expanding colonial involvement.

The prominence of Elizabeth I in the herbal tradition is due in part to her support of the projects of Turner and Lyte and the subsequent influence of those projects in the establishment of the English tradition as discussed earlier in this chapter. Turner's letter "To the most noble and learned Princesse in all kinds of good lerninge / Quene Elizabeth" in the 1568 *First and seconde partes of the Herbal*, dedicates the work of a lifetime under one extensive and sovereign dedicatory epistle. As is the convention in such prefaces, Turner spends the first page expressing his reasons for thus dedicating his work. Left only with the writing of the epistle, he tells the queen that he was in need of "a Patron as had both learning & sufficient autoritie" (sig. *2r). He then relates that in her he finds just such learning, declaring that "I haue both in England / lowe and highe Germanye

---

70 Lena Cowen Orlin, *Private Matters and Public Culture in Post-Reformation England* (Ithaca, New York: Cornell University Press, 1994); Wall, *Staging Domesticity*; and Katharine Gillespie, *Domesticity and Dissent in the Seventeenth Century: English Women Writers and the Public Sphere* (Cambridge: Cambridge University Press, 2004).

71 Gillespie, *Domesticity and Dissent*, 53.

/ and other places of my longe traueil and pelgrimage / neuer spake with any noble or gentle woman that spake so wel and so much congrue fyne & pure Latin" (sig. *2r–*2v), and perceives such supreme authority, writing that "there are none that will denye it [her supreme authority] / sauing onlye the bewitched hipocrites and bound men of the spiritual Babylon" (sig. *2r). Elizabeth thus becomes a paragon not only for her English subjects but also for all of Protestant Europe. In thus setting up the English example, Turner goes on to argue for the primacy of his work, saying that his research precedes or exists outside of those herbals printed on the Continent by Leonhart Fuchs and Pietro Mattioli. Such a defense is necessary in this dedication as he also claims that before his "there was no Englishe Herbal but one al full of vnlearned cacographees and falselye naminge of herbes" (sig. *2v), probably referring to the derivative *Grete Herball* (1516/26). With this volume Turner establishes an English presence in the study of herbs, in England as well as on the Continent. What is more, he does so for the more general profit of England:

> For the knowledge of herbes / trees and shrubbes / is not onelye verye delectable for a Princis minde / but profitable for all the bodies of the Princis hole Realme both to preserue men from sicknes / sorowe and payne that commeth thereby / and also from poison and death / but also necessarye for Phisiciones & apothecaries w^{t}out ye knowlege whereof they can not deuly exercise their office and vocation. . . . (sig. *3r)

Thus Turner's project expresses a sense of emergent English national identity in three ways: first through articulating the exemplar of learning and authority that is Elizabeth; secondly, through establishing an English authority—his own—in herbalism when those in Germany (Fuchs) and Italy (Mattioli) had already done so; finally, in giving to the English people the means "to preserue men from sicknes" (sig.*3r). Elizabeth I, as patron and dedicatee of the work, becomes a source of this proto-nationalistic project at the same time she is a figure for it.[72]

Henry Lyte's dedication to Elizabeth works similarly, yet, given that his is a translation of a French translation of an early Flemish text, the contributions to English national identity made by his project are a bit more difficult to define. Like Turner, Lyte begins his dedicatory epistle providing his reasons for submitting his work to Elizabeth. Like Turner, Lyte first praises Elizabeth's support of education, which encourages scholarship not only through patronage but also in the learning of her subjects, which in turn supports publication in the book's warm reception. Lyte's second reason for thus dedicating his work, however, is tonally different from Turner's. While Turner's praise turns into an expression of anti-Catholic

---

72 See Alix Cooper, *Inventing the Indigenous: Local Knowledge and Natural History in Early Modern Europe* (Cambridge: Cambridge University Press, 2007), and Cathy Shrank, *Writing the Nation in Reformation England, 1530–1580* (Oxford: Oxford University Press, 2004).

sentiment, Lyte's turns into an expression of filial love: "The other [motivation] was that earnest zeale, and feruent desire that I haue, and a long time haue had, to shewe my selfe (by yeelding some fruite of paineful diligence) a thankeful subject to so vertuous a Soueraigne, & a fruitful member of so good a common weale." As the passage develops, Lyte mixes his metaphor of fruitful trees with that of a mother and her children:

> The seconde [motivation] pricketh me continually forwarde with this or the lyke perswasion: That as a thankeful hart towardes a natural mother cannot be better testified, then by loue shewed and practised towardes her dear children: nor a more acceptable fruitfulnesse be required of any one branche, then that which may redounde to the ornament of the whole stocke: so I in no wise should be more able to shewe my thankful minde towardes your highnesse (the most louing and tender mother of this cōmon Weale) then in publishing this historie to ye benefite of your most louing subiectes, as being the best token of loue and diligence that I am at this time able to shew vnto either. (sig. *2r–*2v)

Elizabeth is thus the mother of England to whom Lyte has "shewed and practised" his "love" in translating the herbal for the benefit of her other children.

As it is true that "[d]uring the 1560s and 70s, the image of Elizabeth as mother and nurse of the Church and nation became a commonplace," as Helen Hackett has shown, it is also accurate that Lyte's use of that commonplace has particular effects based on the specificities of his project.[73] Hackett demonstrates that "the figure of the mother . . . signified tender loving care, and as such could be used by subjects to lay claims to rights and privileges," especially when that trope was used in parliamentary or personal petitions.[74] Lyte's comparison of Elizabeth to England's mother, in attesting that he publishes his translation for "the health of many" (sig. *3r), petitions Elizabeth, the patron–mother, to tend to that health through his herbal. While a prayerbook such as Richard Day's *A Booke of Christian Prayers* provides many examples of the figure of Elizabeth as mother in a way that extends the purview of the mother's role to the overseeing of the spiritual well-being of the nation,[75] the claims of Lyte's dedication are much more literal: a mother oversees household health; so shall Elizabeth, England's mother, watch over her nation's physical wellbeing. Whereas Elizabeth herself may manipulate the trope in her marriage speech in order to invoke filial loyalty on the part of her subjects, Lyte's

[73] Helen Hackett, *Virgin Mother, Maiden Queen: Elizabeth I and the Cult of the Virgin Mary* (New York: St. Martin's Press, 1995), 77.

[74] Hackett, *Virgin Mother*, *Maiden Queen*, 77.

[75] Richard Day, *A Booke of Christian Prayers* (London, 1578). For example, in "Another prayer for the church *and all the states thereof, by* John Foxe," we find the following: "thy singular goodnesse hath geuen them a Queéne so calme, so patient, so mercifull: more like a naturall mother then a Princes, to gouern ouer them, such as neither they, nor their auncesters euer read of in the stories of this land before" (sig. H4r).

portrayal of the "louing and tender mother" draws his sovereign's attention to a particular part of her self-asserted role, the mother who cares for a sick child. In sponsoring Lyte's work, Elizabeth attends the sickbeds of all her children, as any mother conceivably would.[76]

Lyte's proto-nationalism is grounded in the vernacular of his project. Unlike Turner, he cannot claim originality in his work or to be the first to write an authentic herbal in English. Instead, his translation of Dodoens makes available in England knowledge formerly known only to the French- and Flemish-speaking peoples. The potential of the vernacular, as Lyte acknowledges it in his address "To the friendly and indifferent Reader," is the widespread availability it provides: "euen the meanest of my Countriemen . . . may yet in time of their necessitie, haue some helpes in their owne, or their neighbours fieldes and gardens at home" (sig. *3r). In this sense, Lyte's figure of Elizabeth I as mother is particularly apt as Lyte's work translates herbal knowledge into English for the general English populace. Unlike Turner, he does not refute or revise or otherwise wrestle with his continental counterparts. His is a project framed in wholly English terms.

The difference between Turner and Lyte's treatment of the herbwife and the witch and their handling of the queen reflects their various intentions for their projects. As a figure for the learned woman, Elizabeth represents a female audience that is well read and thoughtful. As a maternal figure, this female reader uses the herbal only for beneficent ends, in particular for her family. Rather than insecurities, this woman mirrors developing notions of the domestic, those examined by Orlin, Wall, and Gillespie (see n. 70 above), in the dual sense of household and nation. What she does not represent, unlike the herbwife and witch, is one who looks to profit from herbal knowledge. Hers is a charitable practice, one derived from maternal care and economic privilege, thus becoming a model for the practice of the gentlewoman reader.

Lyte's representation of Elizabeth I as mother of England in part informs the ways in which Gerard makes the queen a figurehead. While he does not dedicate his *Herball* to Elizabeth, he does submit it to his employer and patron, William Cecil, "Baron of Burghley, Master of the Court of wardes and Liueries, Chancellor of the Uniuersitie of Cambridge, Knight of the most noble order of the Garter, one of the Lords of hir Maiesties most honorable priuie Counsell, and Lord High Treasurer of England" (sig. A2r). As "one of the Lords of hir Maiesties most honorable priuie Counsell" (sig. A2r) and Elizabeth's chief advisor, Cecil in part serves as representative of the queen, making her an absent presence in the text. This presence is felt in Gerard's herbal from the frontispiece by William Rogers,

[76] Elizabeth I, *Collected Works*, ed. Leah S. Marcus, Janel Mueller, and Mary Beth Rose (Chicago: University of Chicago Press, 2000). The examples from this paragraph follow the suggestions of Helen Hackett's notes, *Virgin Mother, Maiden Queen*, 255 fn. 33–38). A more extensive list of examples of Elizabeth as nurse or mother is indexed in Elkin Calhoun Wilson's *England's Eliza* (Cambridge, Massachusetts: Harvard University Press, 1939).

where Flora reigns in botanical robes, sits on a throne, and arguably wears a floral crown (Figure 1.3). The regal nature of Gerard's Flora is particularly felt when we compare her to her counterpart in Turner's pre-Elizabethan first volume. Turner's Flora is relatively dowdy; her garland is decidedly that, a garland. Rogers determines Flora's relationship to Elizabeth I in the fleur-de-lis she wears around her neck, a flower associated with the English monarchy (in its history with France) through the royal coat-of-arms, reproduced in the left center of the frontispiece.[77] At the same time as the icon of Flora becomes more historical, the historical Elizabeth becomes more iconic.

This iconic Flora–Elizabeth reflects directly the symbolic association of Elizabeth with specific flowers, as discussed at length by Roy Strong and seen most readily in Edmund Spenser's *Shepheardes Calender* and pageants involving the queen. As each flower represented a different virtue (i.e., eglantine equals virginity), Elizabeth, as the aggregate of these virtues, comes to represent the enclosed garden of the Song of Songs. This abstraction, propagated through the gardens of great men like Cecil, moves Elizabeth from the social role of scholar and mother and places her in the position of admired and adored figurehead.[78]

Related to but different from the image of Elizabeth I as mother of England is the regal treatment of Mother Earth found in Gerard. Written to the influential Cecil, Gerard's dedicatory letter might include allusions to royalty, particularly to royal apparel: "For if delight may prouoke mens labour, what greater delight is there than to behold the earth apparelled with plants, as with a robe of imbroidered worke, set with orient pearles, and garnished with great diuersitie of rare and costly iewels" (sig. A2r),[79] later applying this "rare" quality specifically to the gardens of men such as Cecil (sig. A2v). One can imagine Elizabeth in the literal version of such robes; one need think only of Gower's portrait of her.

While royalty appears only in passing in the dedication, the first time Mother Earth enters the prefatory materials, she arguably brings with her much of a female monarch's sense of apparel and pageantry. In the most literary of the prefatory verses, "In commendation of M. Iohn Gerard for his diligence in simpling, by W. Westerman," the author in his first stanza contrasts Gerard with those who "[g]aze . . . vpon the loftie skies, / As rapt with Iunoes painted peacocks traine / When in the aire she vaunts hir Argus eies, / And dips hir bowe in partie-coloured raine" (sig. B3r). This representation of Juno in preparation for Mother Earth to come may draw on the pageant tradition before it; in one of the published progresses

77 The name of the engraver has been discovered by Marjorie Corbett, "The Engraved Title-page to John Gerarde's *Herball or Generall Historie of Plantes*, 1597," *Journal of the Society for the Bibliography of Natural History* 8.3 (1977): 225, who also confirms the identification of the fleur-de-lis, 223.

78 Roy Strong, *The Renaissance Garden in England* (London: Thames and Hudson, 1979), 45–49.

79 Munroe quotes this passage as evidence of the intersections between gardening and embroidery in Munroe, *Gender and the Garden*, 100.

of Elizabeth, that through Norwich, Juno represents and presents (in the form of a jeweled purse) earthly wealth, telling Elizabeth "Thou art beloued of Subjectes farre and nye, / Which is such wealth as money cannot bye" (sig. E1v).[80] Thus the author seems to be contrasting Gerard's pursuits with those monetary pursuits of others. Gerard's is "a lowly course more fitter for his looke" that "doth please him better, than these loftie showes." Gerard is interested in "showes" nonetheless:

> The fruitfull earth he makes his daily booke,
> And turnes such leaues as all his senses knowes:
> He marks the fertill ground whereon he goes,
> And viewes the plentie of our mother Earth,
> Which yeelds supplie against disease and dearth.
>
> Our mother Earth possest with womans pride,
> Perceiuing *Gerard* to be beauties iudge,
> And that hir treasure is not vnespide,
> Of hir faire flowring brats she is no snudge:
> But here and there where *Gerard* loues to trudge,
> Hir verdant mantle spreading round about,
> She boasts the pleasance of hir goodly rout. (sig. B3r)

Not unlike a queen, Mother Earth presents herself so others may look at her, and she appreciates her admirers.

What is more, Gerard's depiction of the earth "set with orient pearles, and garnished with . . . rare and costly iewels" (sig. A2r) and Westerman's images of Gerard as "beauties iudge" and of Earth's "womans pride" (sig. B3r) come from a tradition not strictly herbal. Both Gerard and Westerman draw their imagery from the Petrarchan tradition in the jewel-like features and prideful beauty of the beloved; Gerard is abject to Mother Earth as Astrophil is to Stella (who turns the poet's "gaze" to the "loftie skies," as Westerman avers). That this abject position has political and economic valences has been well proven by literary critics.[81] In having the royally adorned queen-like figure that is Mother Earth show favor to Gerard, Westerman may show Gerard receiving the implied blessing—because of his associations with Cecil—of Elizabeth.

---

[80] In her discussion of the economics of Queen Elizabeth's progresses, Mary Hill Cole relates how some towns "preferred to forgo the expense of a [silver or gilt] cup and instead offer the queen a purse of money," *The Portable Queen: Elizabeth I and the Politics of Ceremony* (Amherst: University of Massachusetts Press, 1999), 101–102.

[81] See Arthur Marotti, "'Love is not love': Elizabethan Sonnet Sequences and the Social Order," *English Literary History* 49.2 (Summer 1982): 396–428, and Ann Rosalind Jones and Peter Stallybrass, "The Politics of *Astrophil and Stella*," *Studies in English Literature, 1550–1900* 24.1 (Winter 1984): 53–68.

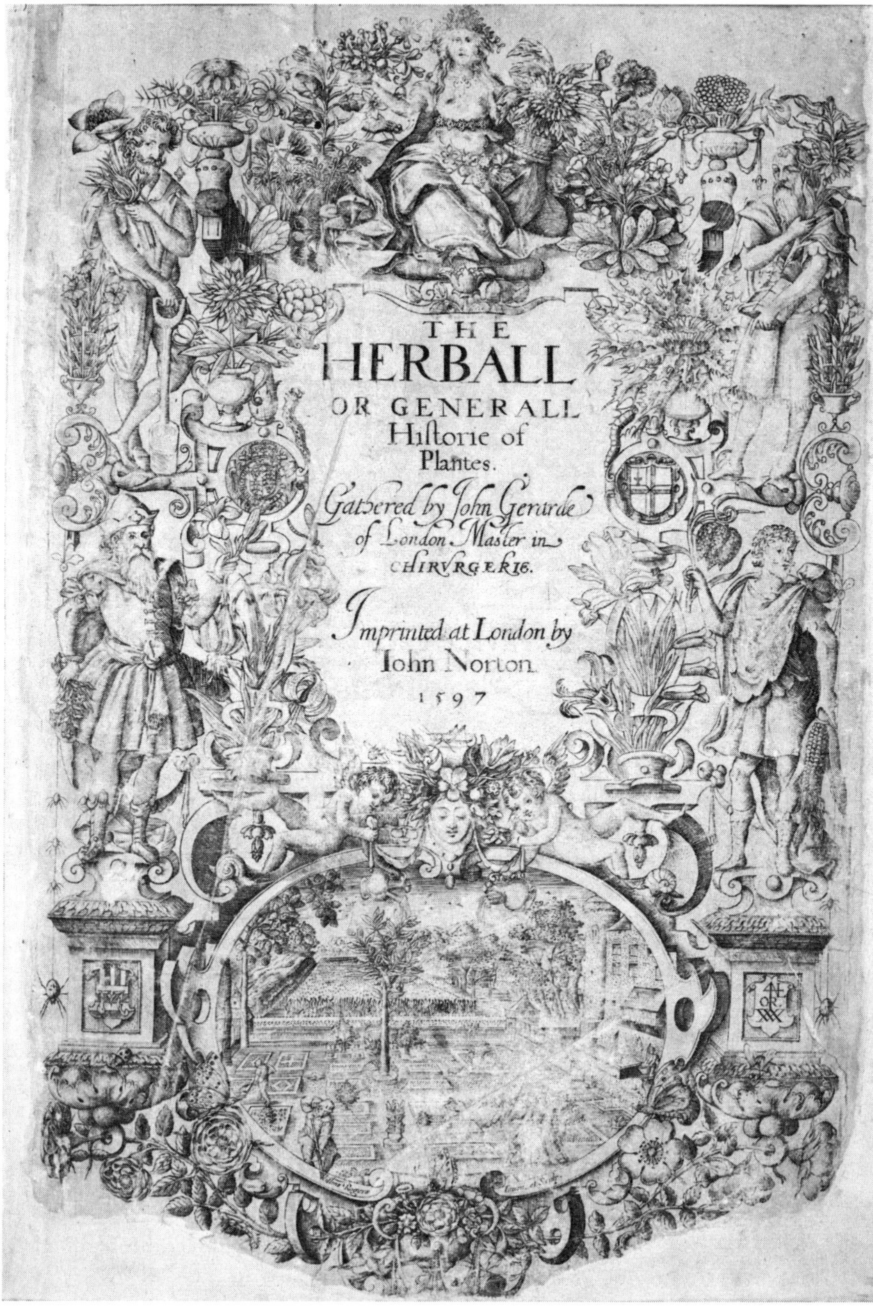

Fig. 1.3 Flora in the frontispiece of Gerard's 1597 *Herball*. Courtesy of the Library of Congress.

Finally, in his address to the reader, the last of the prefatory materials, Gerard writes that he "deuoutly wish[es]" "that most desired benefit of health" "vnto my natiue Countrie, and to the carefull noursing Mother of the same" (n.p.). Given the prevalence of references to Elizabeth as the mother of England discussed with regard to Lyte, the early modern reader would have recognized this "noursing Mother" as Elizabeth I. In such a configuration, Gerard's "noursing Mother" combines with Westerman's "mother Earth"—the earth that earlier in Gerard's address "frankly without violence offereth" plants for human "uses"—and becomes one figure for the English nation. Thus, in Gerard's late Elizabethan herbal, the queen becomes a figurehead for a nation with "New World" interests, reflected in the herbal in the inclusion of such plants as potato and tobacco. She is a figure richly attired and prone to pageantry but also responsible for her nursling England. Whereas Cecil and his garden are the practical movers behind Gerard's herbal, Elizabeth is the spirit behind and above it.

With the seventeenth century, as one would expect, Elizabeth disappears from the mechanisms of patronage and national identity. Johnson's 1633 edition of Gerard, while replicating the prefatory materials of the Elizabethan text, does not feature the regal Flora of the earlier frontispiece. Then, as we have seen, Parkinson dedicates the two volumes of his herbal project to queen-consort Henrietta Maria and King Charles I in the process of gendering different types of herbal authority. Our discussion in this section leads us to consider how, in publishing the project in two phases, Parkinson thus divides the *monarchy* as well as the nature of herbalism. In his addresses to the readership, he splits his plant-based project between flowers and herbs for "delight" and those for "use," dedicating the volume with less medicinal value, the *Paradisus*, to the queen-consort and patroness of the arts, Henrietta Maria, while dedicating the "manlike" *Theatrum* to King Charles, male sovereign, thus gendering and consequently hierarchizing the two halves of the project. How the masculinization of the *Theatrum* has implications for the position of England in New World exploration is reflected in the way in which the female monarch appears in the corners of the *Theatrum*'s frontispiece: four queens representing the continents are dwarfed by Adam and Solomon, images of male Judeo-Christian control of herbal knowledge, in the center. This is not Gerard's Flora who reigns over the male figures beneath her. The female monarch represented in Parkinson's works is either the Catholic wife of the new—not yet embattled—king or the representative of the lands submitting to English conquest.

Gone are the references to Mother Earth and Elizabeth, mother of England. Here is the *kingly* male provider: "For as your Majesty is *Summus Pater patriae* … that not onely provideth for their soules health, that they may have the pure Word of God . . . but many wayes also for their bodily estates . . . that every one may live obediently and peaceably under their owne Vine and Figtree" ("To the Kings Most Excellent Maiestie," n.p.). Reminding us of Parkinson's obsessions with patrilineage, Charles I is "*Pater patriae*," literally the "father of the fatherland." Such a dedication during the early years of the English religious wars asserts not only Parkinson's sense of indebtedness, but also his political position with regard to the absolutist monarch confronted by religious conflict. Parkinson's dedication is not so much a work reflecting proto-nationalistic translation and appropriation of knowledge, as it is one that asserts British monarchical power in the face of colonial expansion and increasing domestic strife.

The implications of this historical difference may become clearer through the ways in which Parkinson introduces Queen Elizabeth I in various entries throughout his *Theatrum Botanicum*, which do not hold her up as paragon of learning or icon of the English nation. Given that the work was published two generations after Elizabeth's death, it is surprising that we see her at all. The first time she appears in Parkinson's herbal, in the entry on bryony, the queen lies on her deathbed: "it is most usually being made into powder taken in wine, or if any refuse that manner, the roote may be boyled either in a little broth, (as it was to Queene *Elizabeth* in her last sickenesse, without her consent or sence in the taste) or wine" (181). Not only is Elizabeth I sick and weak, but also she is being obstinate and consequently deceived by her caregivers. This is not the learned and authoritative Elizabeth of Lyte and Turner. She is vulnerable to both illness and intrigue.

The next time she appears in the *Theatrum*, it is in the entry on "*Vlmaria sive Regina prati*. Medowsweete or Medesweete"; the Latin *Regina prati* (Queen of the meadow) Parkinson—unlike Gerard (886)—has left untranslated in his heading. In the entry, Parkinson relates that "Queene *Elizabeth* of famous memory did more desire [meadowsweet] then any other sweet herbe to strew her Chambers withall" (593).[82] This depiction, while diverting, presents an Elizabeth much more akin to Parkinson's portrayal of Henrietta Maria in the *Paradisus*, a queen who "much delighted with all the faire Flowers of a Garden" (sig. **2r), than of the sovereign Charles in the *Theatrum*, "chiefe of [his] people under God" (n.p.). The meadowsweet entry limits her powers while relegating the queen to the realm of delight. She is not in the privy chamber conferring with her counselors but rather in her bedchamber relaxing with her servingmaids.

The final mention of Elizabeth is not of her but of her physicians. I quote the entry on "the Boxe tree" at length because the entire passage paints a portrait of an age less worthy of pride than that found in the sixteenth-century volumes:

> The leaves of box are hot and dry, and astringent withall, as the taste declareth, and therefore assuredly doth dry and binde, yet is it not much used in Physicke by any now adayes that I know . . . *Fernelius* onely doth number the leaves hereof among those things that doe purge, but the practise thereof is worne out of use, yet I remember that Doctor *Smith*, that was one of Queene *Elizabeths* Physitions, appointed the decoction of an ounce of the leaves of Boxe for a purging medicine, to be boyled in whey, and a dramme of the pouther in broth. But *Matthiolus* contesteth against such as tooke it . . . . (1429)

82 Quoted in Rohde, *Old English Herbals*, 162.

This record of the faults of "Doctor Smith" shows how this is not praise of a contemporary but rather a disparaging look at the ignorance of past times. One need only remember Turner's pained recollection of the "vnlearned cacographees" of the previous English herbals and the "ignorance in simples" at the time he began his studies to comprehend the reasons for Parkinson's criticism. Parkinson's is not the first herbal in English, but in an attempt to make up for his belatedness, he paints a picture of an ignorant past in part to signify his advancements. In line with our previous discussion, the disparagement of the Elizabethan age found in the entry on boxtree may also be personal; the rivalry Parkinson feels with regard to Gerard because of the 1633 and 1636 re-editions of Gerard's herbal is often palpable in the *Theatrum*. "Doctor Smith" may be a stand-in for another of "Queene Elizabeths Physitions," Lancelot Brown, whose commendatory letter comes directly after Gerard's dedication to Cecil, a letter replicated in the later editions. In sum, unlike the dedications to Elizabeth that praise the climate of learning in that time, Parkinson's entry on boxtree shows a backward Elizabethan age.

It should be clear that none of these examples from Parkinson holds up Elizabeth as an authoritative sovereign. On the contrary, they seem to degrade—at the very least restrict—the queen by depicting her as frivolous or weak. In part what may inform this characterization is the gender politics of the period, the emphasis on "patriarchal authority" against the "deified" virgin, first fostered by Charles I's father, James I.[83] Parkinson creates a "delicate" or "dainty" Elizabeth—both in the sense of "fastidiousness" and that of a poor constitution.[84] This depiction coincides with his "Garden of Pleasant Flowers," the *Paradisus*, but also with other entries in the *Theatrum*, which describe "[o]ur daintiest women" who "doe put [marjoram] to still among their other sweet hearbs, to make sweet washing water" (14), or women who need herbs in their frail health as in the entry on rest harrow: "as daintie a medicine for tender stomacks as any the daintiest Lady in the Land can desire to take, being troubled with any the aforesaid greifes" (995). In the entries that depict her, Elizabeth becomes one with all women—particularly ladies—in the text, who use herbs only for toilet or the relief of their own discomforts, rarely in the care of others.

Indeed, there are only isolated mentions in Parkinson's *Theatrum* of women who tend to the health of others: "the women of *Bury* in *Suffolke*" (856) who use pepperwort in their midwifery, the "men and women leeches"—"the vulgar sort"—who use parsley to "provoke urine" (449) and "any good Gentlewoman in the land, that would do good either to her owne family, or other her poore neighbors" with a salve made of bugle (526). Women are public practitioners in only circumscribed—or "vulgar"—contexts. In the "manlike worke" of the

---

83 Linda Levy Peck, *The Mental World of the Jacobean Court* (Cambridge: Cambridge University Press, 1991), 7.

84 "dainty, a^5 and a^7," *Oxford English Dictionary*, http://dictionary.oed.com/cgi/entry/50057167.

Theatrum, Parkinson's intent, even in these mentions, seems to be to downplay female authority. In depicting a "dainty" Elizabeth, one with a refined sense of smell and who is tended to by others, not the "Mother of England" who tends to the health of an entire nation through Protestant vigilance, Parkinson reflects the general glorification of male authority he has undertaken in this work.

As I hope this chapter has helped to illuminate, Parkinson's impetus to thus limit or downplay women's medical authority may have more to do with his own professional "insecurities" because of associations with female practice and his late position in the tradition than with practical realities. While he limits women's practice within the confines of charity and the home, Parkinson's predecessor Gerard (more secure in his position under Cecil) praises Anne Wilbraham for her knowledge in the art of healing, albeit, again, among "hir poore neighbours" (315). As we will see, moreover, female writers themselves, who conceivably took up the pen from within these limits, worked to expand them and demonstrated their capacity around them, and often women accomplished the expansion of their authority—whether in medical or writing practice—through *owning an herbal*. The irony that as many as four of the female-owned texts discussed in Chapter 2 are copies of the *Theatrum Botanicum* should challenge any assumptions we would make about the uses of the texts.

In assessing the role of Elizabeth I in *Theatrum*, however, it is important to remember that even though she may become the conventional dainty lady in Parkinson's book, she is not simply any woman; she is "Queene Elizabeth of famous memory." If we consider recent analyses of the representations of Elizabeth in Stuart England, we come to realize that there is most likely something specifically political going on in Parkinson's depiction of the virgin queen. Take, for example, Christopher Hill's long list of texts that support his claim that "a favourite method of political denigration within acceptable limits was to praise Queen Elizabeth—often excessively—in order by implication to criticize her successors," to which researchers in the field of women writers have added the examples of Diana Primrose's *A Chaine of Pearl* (1630) and Anne Bradstreet's paean to Elizabeth (1650).[85] While in these instances Charles I may be critiqued

[85] Christopher Hill, "Censorship and English Literature," *The Collected Essays of Christopher Hill, Volume I: Writing and Revolution in 17th Century England* (Amherst: University of Massachusetts Press, 1985), 57; on Primrose, Kari Boyd McBride, "Contextual Materials for 'A Chaine of Pearl' by Diana Primrose," Introductions to Works, *Renaissance Women Online*, Women Writers Project, Brown University, http://textbase.wwp.brown.edu/WWO/php/rInt.php?doc=rInt.00272.html (accessed March 2, 2009), and on Bradstreet, John Watkins, *Representing Elizabeth in Stuart England: Literature, History, and Sovereignty* (Cambridge: Cambridge University Press, 2002), 101–107. See also Lisa Gim, "'Faire *Eliza's* Chaine': Two Female Writers' Literary Links to Queen Elizabeth I," *Maids and Mistresses, Cousins and Queens: Women's Alliances in Early Modern England*, ed. Susan Frye and Karen Robertson (New York: Oxford University Press, 1999), 183–98, and Elizabeth H. Hageman and Katherine Conway, eds., *Resurrecting Elizabeth I in*

through praise of Elizabeth, what we may find in Parkinson is the counterpoint; in a work dedicated to Charles that calls him "*Summus Pater patriae*," the weakening and containment of a previous monarch, a monarch who has been held up as a paragon of Protestant leadership by the king's critics, have the opposite function: they to counteract the critiques.

More probing examinations of Elizabeth's representational role in Stuart England help us to see the intricacies in these depictions. In light of John Watkins's reading of "Tacitean narrations of the Elizabethan past,"[86] especially that by William Camden, Elizabeth on her sickbed as seen in the bryony entry becomes an image of a weak monarch reliant on her robust—and deceptive—counselors.[87] The Elizabeth taking delight in flowers is thus connected with Henrietta Maria of the *Paradisus*, a link Watkins finds in other royalist depictions of Elizabeth as a means of deflecting Protestant critiques away from the Catholic queen.[88] While the overt meanings of these passages are about medicine and meadowsweet, the political context of Stuart England infuses this treatment of the queen with court intrigue and religious tension. And Parkinson's rivalry with Gerard thus takes added significance as well, as the disparagement of the Elizabethan age has more than personal implications.

That this kind of politicking occurs in an herbal may baffle the twenty-first-century reader, but many in and around the study of botany are demonstrating that the history of plants and of botanical knowledge has much to do with the workings of culture in general. Historians such as Alix Cooper have shown us how the delineation of "indigenous" plants reflects issues of regional identity and reactions to colonial expansion.[89] Londa Schiebinger has demonstrated recently how the transmission of one plant—and of the kinds of knowledge about that plant—mirrors much larger cultural currents than one would at first expect.[90] Antonio Barrera discusses the uses of "local herbs" in Spanish colonization,[91] and Deborah Harkness has shown us the interactions of collaboration, competition, and xenophobia as they inform botanical study in early modern London.[92] Considering

Seventeenth-Century England (Madison, New Jersey: Fairleigh Dickinson University Press, 2007).

86 Watkins, *Representing Elizabeth*, 56.

87 Watkins, *Representing Elizabeth*, 58–68. See also R. Malcolm Smuts, *Court Culture and the Origins of a Royalist Tradition in Early Stuart England* (Philadelphia: University of Pennsylvania Press, 1987), 26, and Patrick Collinson, "William Camden and the Anti-Myth of Elizabeth: Setting the Mould?" in *The Myth of Elizabeth*, ed. Susan Doran and Thomas S. Freeman (Basingstoke, Hampshire: Palgrave Macmillan, 2003), 79–98.

88 Watkins, *Representing Elizabeth*, 91–92.

89 Cooper, *Inventing the Indigenous*.

90 Schiebinger, *Plants and Empire*.

91 Antonio Barrera, "Local Herbs, Global Medicines: Commerce, Knowledge, and Commodities in Spanish America," *Merchants and Marvels*, 163–81.

92 Harkness, *The Jewel House*, 15–56.

how the early English herbals present the knowledge of plants, particularly those plants that are English, in proto-nationalistic terms, it makes sense that later herbals would also register when that domestic arena is on shakier ground. The treatment of the queen in these herbals proves to be just such a case. So even at the same time the queen may reflect the role of the gentlewoman practitioner, that role becomes inflected by the political climate surrounding it.

While the female herbal practitioner was very much a historical reality, her presence in the early modern vernacular English herbal is evidence of much more than her social role. Her presence in these volumes reveals to us the anxieties and conflicts surrounding the publication of herbal texts and allows us to see the stages in the development of the English print herbal tradition as those anxieties and conflicts mutate or dissolve. Close examination of these changes over the century between Turner and Parkinson reveals that these folios illuminate some aspects of the history of herbal practice, but they tell us more—obviously—about the history of herbal texts and the construction of the female herbal reader. We will examine another aspect of print herbal history, the owning and reading of herbals by women, in the following chapters. In considering herbals as objects owned and read by women, we find that female practitioners are no longer metaphor, metonym, or icon but rather various, dynamic, and multi-dimensional.

Chapter 2
Inscriptions in Herbal Texts and the Location of Medical Authority

As we have come to see the way that the English herbal tradition increasingly acknowledged the gentlewoman reader—at the same time that it may have sought to delimit her practice—we now turn to the numerous instances in which we can determine that women owned these same volumes. Specifically, cases of early modern women's ownership of the authoritative herbals by William Turner, Rembert Dodoens, John Gerard, and John Parkinson examined in the previous chapter serve as our subjects of inquiry in this chapter. By "ownership" I mean not only the material possession of an item within the household but also the claim to the knowledge held in the book. In asserting ownership, women positioned the volume within the household, potentially articulating their role within that household as healer. They did not subscribe only to the uses of herbs designated for women: all of the textual knowledge was open before the women who owned the herbals. These women were as likely to use rue to stop a nosebleed as to end a pregnancy, and while Anne Wilbraham's cure for the ague using docks discussed in Chapter 1 is available to them, John Bennet's much more aggressive treatment resided on the same page. And even though the learned gentlewoman with a charitable practice was the female reader preferred by the herbal author, any woman with English literacy and the requisite moneys could own this knowledge. The nature of these books as volumes to be used determined that these women did not own the herbals simply for their own solitary edification. In signifying ownership of an authoritative herbal, these women also gave evidence of the various "social networks" to which they belonged and the cultural influences to which they were subject.[1] Herbal ownership thus proves to mean many things across households and between individuals, and delineating the variations between the examples of ownership further demonstrates how Englishwomen's herbal texts may point to social variables and individual realities beyond a general and monolithic medical practice by women.

This chapter has as its foundation more than twenty examples of herbal ownership before or around 1700, which are evidenced by life-writings, wills, inventories, and artworks, along with fifteen early modern inscriptions in the actual

---

[1] Heidi Brayman Hackel also uses this phrase, *Reading Material in Early Modern England: Print, Gender, and Literacy* (Cambridge: Cambridge University Press, 2005), 219; Mary Erler discusses "the lives and networks" of the woman reader, *Women, Reading, and Piety in Late Medieval England* (Cambridge: Cambridge University Press, 2002), 6.

volumes (see Appendix B). It is the last of these that provides a more specific focus here, as these fragments introduce some of the wider social implications at play in more extensive works. While some of the analysis may seem speculative, I hope to show how the interplay between signatures, patterns across various texts, supporting biographical documents, and contexts provided by more sustained engagements with the herbal text all make fragments more than incomplete. After having uncovered some of the social implications behind these inscriptions in this chapter, in Chapter 3 I approach three longer manuscripts written by women before 1650: Lady Margaret Hoby's diary from 1599 to 1605, Lady Grace Mildmay's early seventeenth-century textual remains, and Elizabeth Isham's book inventory (c. 1648) and autobiography (early 1640s), all of which record the possession of and reading of an herbal. I mention this now as throughout the analysis of the inscriptions, I will be anticipating the extended works of these three women because the social contexts implicit in the signatures may be more broadly realized in the life-writings. Nonetheless, for now, the inscriptions in and of themselves have much to tell us.

For the purpose of analysis I have had to loosen my date restrictions to include inscriptions in the late seventeenth and possibly early eighteenth centuries (yet only considering ownership of books printed before 1650). I have done so because the comparative analysis I would like to perform requires a sizable group and the later date allows for more owners of the seventeenth-century Gerard editions and the 1640 *Theatrum Botanicum* (of which there are more extant examples) to be included in that comparison. More and varied examples also allow us to explore better the different meanings of that ownership. In attempting to limit my examples to within a century of the books' publication dates, I have tried to keep them outside of antiquarian collections such as the 1597 Gerard once owned by the modernist poet Hilda Doolittle (known as H.D.) found at Beinecke Library;[2] a modern book plate adds the possibility that the owner is a collector rather than someone who is interested in the book's contents for their use value. In supporting my analysis of fifteen herbal inscriptions with other kinds of evidence of ownership, I show how the inscriptions belong to a larger complex of texts.

Before embarking upon extensive comparative analysis, I turn to an illustrative example (and the first identifiable signature in my research adventure) found in an uncatalogued provenance in Henry Lyte's 1578 translation of Dodoens's *Crŭijdeboeck*, *A Nievve Herball*, at the Yale Medical Historical Library.[3] The

---

2 John Gerard, *The Herball or Generall Historie of Plantes* (1597), Beinecke Si8 0168.

3 Rembert Dodoens, *A Nievve Herball, or Historie of Plantes*, trans. Henry Lyte (London, 1578), Yale Medical Historical Library, Herbal Collection. Much of the following information has been presented in Rebecca Laroche, "Elizabeth Bagot's Herbal," *Yale University Library Gazette*, 81.1–2 (2006 October): 21–26, and developed further, as was the section on Anne Purefoy below, in Laroche, "'To take in hand the practise of phisick': Early Modern Women's Signatures in Print Medical Texts," in *New Ways of Looking at Old*

signature "Elizabeth: Bagot" appears in the bottom margin of this particular title page (Figure 2.1). Elizabeth Bagot's signature—not confident, as the hand has crossed out one "B" and replaced it with one better executed—is most definitively that of Elizabeth Cave Bagot (d. 1638), child of Roger and Elizabeth Cecil Cave. Through her mother, she is also the niece of the royal minister Lord Burghley, William Cecil (1520/21–1598).[4] Cecil is most notable as close advisor to Elizabeth I, but it is also important for us to recognize again, as discussed in Chapter 1, that he was also famous for his gardens, and his gardener, John Gerard, dedicated his herbal to him in 1597. This familial connection to Gerard's *Herball* suggests—as anyone of the Cecil clan would likely prefer a text with such ties—that Lyte's translation was purchased before the publication of the later text and that the signature may have been written in the herbal before 1597.

This date is entirely possible because Elizabeth Cave was married to Walter Bagot (c. 1557–1623) of Staffordshire in 1586, and in a point to be analyzed later in this chapter, her hesitation in writing "Bagot" suggests that the name may be new to her pen.[5] We know much about her husband Walter and his extended family because of the correspondence and private papers in the Bagot collection kept at the Folger Shakespeare Library. Through the correspondence found there, we know that his siblings often called on Walter Bagot to use his political and financial influence to help them weather various domestic and social tempests, and we know that Walter and Elizabeth experienced the untimely death of their son Lewis in his young adulthood. It is also through this collection that we can identify without doubt the Elizabeth Bagot in Yale's *Nievve Herball* as the wife of Walter, because this collection holds one letter with a signature nearly identical (the herbal's "Elizabeth:" abbreviated to "Eliz:" in the letter) to the one penned in that book.[6]

The letter is an appealing example of familiar correspondence. Dated the 7th of July, 1614, Elizabeth's missive accompanies documents that Walter has requested be sent to him while he is away attending to business in London. The letter's body is written in a hand that does not seem to be Elizabeth's, being most likely that of a household secretary; only the roman hand of the signature bears resemblance to

---

Texts IV, ed. Michael Denbo (Tempe, Arizona: Renaissance English Text Society, 2009), 269–78.

4 M. W. Greenslade, "Bagot Family," *Oxford Dictionary of National Biography*, Online Version (Oxford: Oxford University Press, 2004–06), http://www.oxforddnb.com/view/article/71871 (accessed July 27, 2007).

5 Greenslade, "Bagot Family."

6 Elizabeth Bagot, "Letter," Folger Manuscript L.a.48. For a reproduction, transcription, and brief analysis of this letter, see Rebecca Laroche, "Gendering Hands, Gendering Business: A Letter from Elizabeth Bagot," http://www.folger.edu/html/folger_institute/mm/EssayRL.html (accessed July 25, 2007). My thanks to Heather Wolfe and Steven May for their help in transcribing this letter.

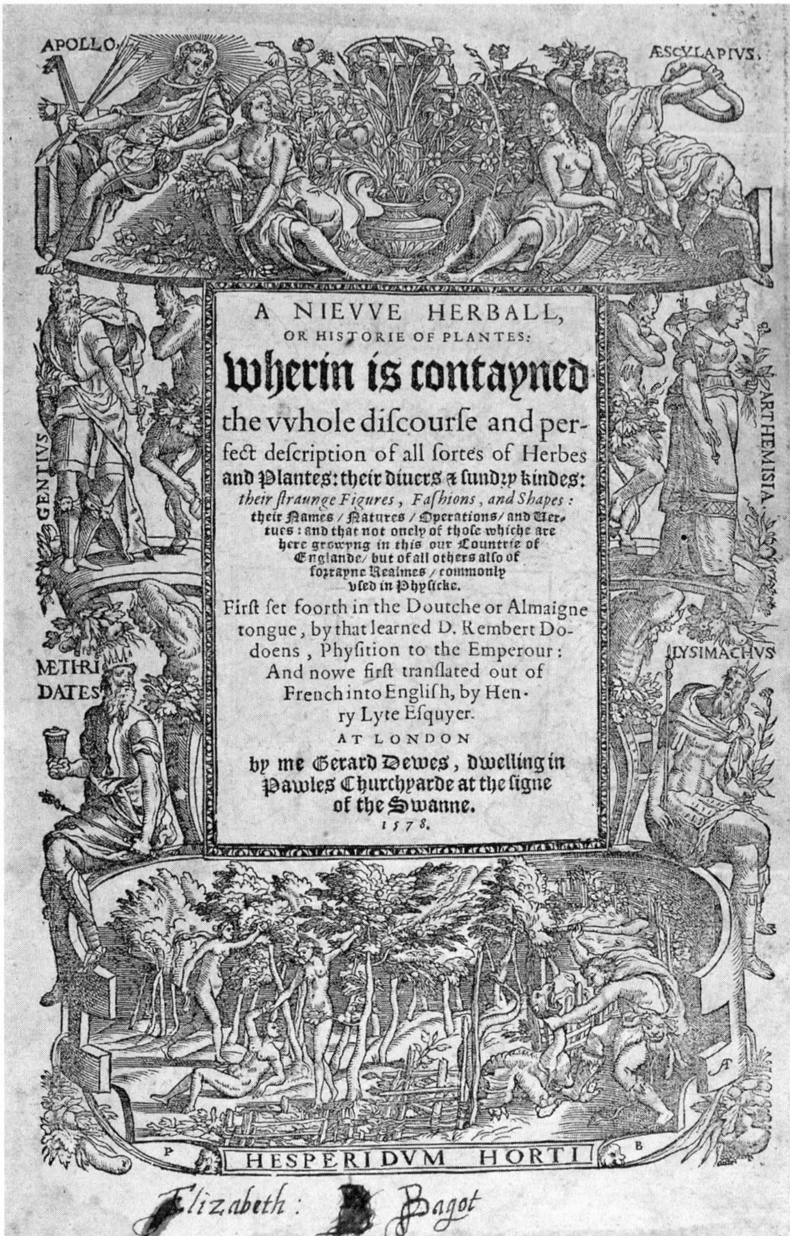
A NIEVVE HERBALL,
OR HISTORIE OF PLANTES:
wherin is contayned
the vvhole diſcourſe and perfect deſcription of all ſortes of Herbes and Plantes: their diuers & ſundry kindes: *their ſtraunge Figures, Faſhions, and Shapes:* their Names, Natures, Operations, and Vertues: and that not onely of thoſe whiche are here growyng in this our Countrie of Englande, but of all others alſo of forrayne Realmes, commonly vſed in Phyſicke.
Firſt ſet foorth in the Doutche or Almaigne tongue, by that learned D. Rembert Dodoens, Phyſition to the Emperour: And nowe firſt tranſlated out of French into Engliſh, by Henry Lyte Eſquyer.
AT LONDON
by me Gerard Dewes, dwelling in Pawles Churchyarde at the ſigne of the Swanne.
1578.

Fig. 2.1 Elizabeth Bagot's signature signifying ownership. 1578 Dodoens, Yale Medical Historical Library, Herbal+. By permission of Yale University, Harvey Cushing/John Hay Whitney Medical Library.

that of the Yale inscription. The letter tells us that she has been searching for items in her husband's study:

> My good Watt; I haue receiued yor l[ett]re, and giue god thankes for your good health; and safety in yor iorney. You wrytt to me to sende you a blacke boxe of wrytinges, which I haue sent you by this bearer hauinge in it these p[ar]cells, 2 ffynes, one ffeoffm[en]t and one examplificac[i]on, wch I founde at Blythfeilde my self in your studie this day, and by chaunce knew them withou[t any] helpe. . . . For our frendes in these p[ar]tes, and the state of our busynes . . . here, I referre to the reporte of this bearer.

This letter confirms what we also glean from Walter's extensive correspondence: during their marriage, Walter was often away from their home in Staffordshire. As we see here and in many women's letter collections from the period, Elizabeth, as female head, took care of the household business in his absence.[7] In her closing, she goes on to refer to "yo[u]r busynesse" in London, but in the body of the letter she alludes to "our busynes," the shared management of the Staffordshire estate. The context of the household remote from London is an important one for the purchase of the herbal in the first decade of their marriage. As female head of household, Bagot oversaw household health and accounts ("our busynes"), and it was in this capacity that she attained a copy of *A Nievve Herball*. She did so for an immediate reference book regarding household illness and injury and as a matter of thrift in household expense. Indeed, as we remember from our previous chapter's discussion, it was translator Henry Lyte who promised that his reader may "in time of their necessitie, haue some helpes in their owne, or their neighbours fieldes and gardens at home."[8] With herbal erudition at her fingertips, she was able to forgo the expense of the physician in less urgent cases.

The existence of Elizabeth Bagot's letter allows us to give a background and history—however brief—to what would otherwise be just a signature, but I am most interested here in what the signature itself can tell us. In writing her name,

---

[7] Letters by women that show the role of the female head of household in the absence of London-bound husbands can be found in the following collections: Brilliana Harley, *Letters of the Lady Brilliana Harley, Wife of Sir Robert Harley, of Brampton Bryan, Knight of Bath*, ed. and intro. Thomas Taylor Lewis, A. M., vicar of Bridstow, Herefordshire (London: Camden Society, 1854); Maria Thynne, "Letters," in *Lay by Your Needles Ladies, Take the Pen: Writing Women in England, 1500–1700*, ed. Suzanne Trill, Kate Chedgzoy, and Melanie Osborne, 76–78 (London: St. Martin's Press, 1997); Countess of Huntingdon, Elizabeth Hastings (1597–1633), *Correspondence*, Huntington Library, Hastings Collection.

[8] Henry Lyte, "To the friendly and indifferent Reader," in Dodoens, *A Nievve Herball*, sig.*3r.

Bagot claimed her ownership of a relatively expensive volume.[9] She also owned a certain level of literacy, one that could not be taken for granted among even England's elite women. Most importantly, with this signature, she also claims ownership of a certain kind of knowledge. By signing the volume, Elizabeth Bagot claims the role of healer, at least in her household, and, with this role, she takes part in the medical authority articulated in the pages of the herbal.

That is, in writing her signature, Elizabeth Bagot does not write her name only along the entries related to domestic care. She writes her name in a prominent position on the title page, making the entire book her own. The presence of her signature thus destabilizes any gendering of medical authority that may occur in the volume itself (though Lyte's paratextual elements are less aggressive in doing so than Parkinson's). Bagot signs her name to the knowledge of Dodoens, not simply to the iconic representations of Queen Artemisia or the Fates on the title page or to the dedication to the female sovereign. The text exists in lieu of the Flemish physician as the gentlewoman practices in the absence (either by economy or geography) of a physician's care.[10] This insight will be most important in understanding the relationship between the previous chapter on male-authored herbals and the two following this one, which are dedicated to extended writings by women. The woman's signature signifies the space between reading (the prelude to practice) and practice (which in turn may be recorded in writing). It signifies the ownership of the text.

The variety of social situations in which a woman articulates herbal knowledge and practice through ownership should not be underestimated. A woman may come to herbal ownership as a newly married woman or even in girlhood, only to leave that herbal behind in her widowhood. She may be the first owner or the fourth, a circumstance that changes the economic signification of the text. She may come to own the herbal through inheritance, but that inheritance may as well come from a male relation or family friend as from a mother. She may own the book as a female head of household, but the female head may be either unmarried or married, may have ten children or none. Each of these contexts implies something different about a woman's relationship to the authoritative medical text as well as to the community surrounding her. So many social contexts, moreover, entail that a given woman may relate to established medical authority in any number of fashions. This last concept will be more fully realized in the case studies in the third chapter, where the authors read the herbal in conjunction with, in the absence

---

9 On the relative cost for various volumes in the period, see Francis Johnson, "Notes on English Retail Book-Prices, 1550–1640," *The Library* 5.5 (1950–51): 83–112.

10 Ian Mortimer argues that physicians were more readily available than previously assumed, but this does not diminish women's roles in immediate or pre-physician care or in instances when area physicians were otherwise overextended; Ian Mortimer, "The Rural Medical Marketplace in Southern England c. 1570–1720," in *Medicine and the Market in England and Its Colonies, c. 1450–c. 1850*, ed. Mark S. R. Jenner and Patrick Wallis (Basingstoke, Hampshire: Palgrave Macmillan, 2007), 69–87.

of, or as resistance to, the authority of a physician, but we can begin to see here in the simple signing of a name how ownership of the herbal's textual medical authority is not simply a capitulation to the medical hierarchies that some of the herbal authors espouse and may indeed problematize those authorial assertions.

"Her Booke": Women's Inscriptions in Folio Herbals

Identifying the woman behind the signature of Elizabeth Bagot convinced me that such inscriptions might be worth pursuing, and soon I found that many other libraries, often medical historical archives, offered such a signature, sometimes two. Not that I have been able to identify everyone behind the signatures, but I have been able to discover many signatures that have markers of early modernity: a colon at the end of a name, a secretary "e," a long "s," the spelling of "boock" and "booke," or the presence of "y^{e}." Others are explicitly seventeenth-century: "Jane Baker 1660," "Mes Anne Whitehall of Yildersley her booke 1672," "Mary Saltonstall 1674," "Mary Chambers her book amen. 1689," the wife of John F. who died in 1672, and Anne Purefoy's gift from her sister recorded in 1643.[11] Even without dates, as in the example of Bagot above and those of Sarah Gibson and Katherine Shirley discussed below, biographical details have helped to place inscriptions in a moment before 1700. My continuing search for these signatures has been in part inspired by the groundbreaking work of Mary Erler, whose quest for signs of early modern women's ownership of devotional incunabula has brought women to light who previously were beyond our imagining.[12] I hope that the women rediscovered through these herbals may similarly bring a new understanding to women's reading and writing practices and that the complex of texts and contexts may continue to be expanded as new signatures and new associations emerge.

The rest of my analysis will closely examine some of the more suggestive examples of the inscriptions, but I first would like to raise the possibility that each woman conceivably had different motivations for writing her name in these volumes and that all of them wrote their names with an implied sense of audience: someone in the future of the book was meant to see the individual's signature. Both Heidi Brayman Hackel and William Sherman have looked into and provided evidence for different reasons for writing one's name, and my discussion here

[11] The examples of signatures listed can be found at the Academy of Natural Sciences, University of Pennsylvania, Texas A&M, the Linnaean Society Library, the Library of Congress, the Folger Shakespeare Library respectively. See Appendix B for the list of examples and call numbers. An earlier version of this list appears in Laroche, "'To take in hand the practise of phisick,'" 272–73. My thanks to Karen Reeds for telling me about the Linnaean Society copy.

[12] Erler, *Women, Reading, and Piety*.

looks to extend their analysis and specify it in the context of herbal ownership.[13] The woman who wrote her name may have articulated her position in a lineage, either coming after a previous owner or looking toward posterity, or in more overt examples, usually found in a Bible, she could be recording a family history.[14] In a related manner, her signature could be distinguishing her library from the larger family collection.[15] As in the instance of Elizabeth Franklin and Anne Purefoy discussed below, the signature may have been meant to mark a specific occasion, in their case, the bestowal of a gift. With regard to the particular nature of the herbal, a signature could also designate a woman's position in the larger society: the mark of ownership of a folio herbal demonstrated that she and her family could afford such a volume; furthermore, the signature was meant to keep a valuable object from being purloined (as fanciful examples cited by Brayman Hackel record), or the inscriber may have been lending the book and expecting its return.[16] Finally, as posited with Elizabeth Bagot, a woman may have written her name in an herbal to articulate her position in the household as one who had medical knowledge, especially against others who may not have had such expertise. While it is the woman's participation in the attainment and circulation of medical knowledge that will come to most interest us in the final chapters, in the end, the reason(s) may have been for any one or any combination of the above (or others not yet thought of). Importantly, moreover, the majority of these motivations have pointed to some sort of social group.[17] Even when the signer is attempting to establish individual privilege against the group, the group's presence has been at least implied. The ownership of an herbal is doubly marked in its social positioning, as medicine inevitably involves others.

The four examples of autographs or inscriptions to be examined in the body of this chapter, along with others that support my readings of them, refer directly to the occasion for writing and point indirectly to the network surrounding the inscriber. A husband's elegy found in a copy of Parkinson's *Theatrum Botanicum*,

---

13 Brayman Hackel, *Reading Material*; William Sherman, *Used Books: Marking Readers in Renaissance England* (Philadelphia: University of Pennsylvania Press, 2008).

14 Sherman, *Used Books*, 59–60.

15 Paul Morgan, "Frances Wolfreston and 'Hor Bouks': A Seventeenth-Century Woman Book-Collector," *The Library* 6.2 (1989): 201. Rebecca Laroche, "Catherine Tollemache's Library," *Notes and Queries* 251.2 (June 2006): 157–58, and Laroche, "To take in hand the practise of phisick." See also Brayman Hackel, *Reading Material*, 214–15.

16 Brayman Hackel, *Reading Material*, 218. For a discussion of book prices in the period, see Johnson, "Notes on English Retail Book-Prices."

17 This insight is related to that of Natalie Zemon Davis's that the book is a "carrier of relationships," Natalie Zemon Davis, "Printing and the People," *Society and Culture in Early Modern France* (Stanford: Stanford University Press, 1975), 192, as quoted in William Sherman, "What Did Renaissance Readers Write in Their Books?" in *Books and Readers in Early Modern England: Material Studies*, ed. Jennifer Andersen and Elizabeth Sauer (Philadelphia: University of Pennsylvania Press), 126.

an eighteenth-century provenance in a 1633 Gerard, a gift from an elder sister to a younger one of the multipurpose *Paradisus Terrestris*, and a girl's handwriting practice in a 1578 Dodoens all bear with them some sense of the book as an object as well as an occasion for reading and writing. The names recorded in these examples also do not exist in isolation; that is, other names or signatures exist alongside those of the female owner, suggesting in the juxtaposition the social relationships to which I have referred. Some of the inscriptions I would like to consider closely are written by men, because it is through the cohabitation of signatures, regardless of gender, that we can learn most about these ownerships. Through the implied social contexts surrounding the women's ownership signatures, we may also learn more about where female herbal authority is located and how it is established or, alternatively, how it is fluid in its constructions. Of course, the book eventually leaves the hands of the female owner, and it is the nature of the inscription that determines how her ownership of medical knowledge will or will not be remembered. The first example under our scrutiny best illuminates the memorialization such signatures embody.

Authority *in Memoriam*

The Library of Congress's second copy of John Parkinson's *Theatrum Botanicum* contains the following poem (sonnet-like in rhyme scheme if not in meter) on the blank verso after the front matter (Figure 2.2):

> Reader, behold, & weepe; This Tombe,
>   Which keepes this sacred Dust, containes,
> though crouded in a Narrow Roome
>   More Worth then in the World Remaines./
>
> What progresse hath thy blessed Soule
>   Made since it Left the breathles clay?
> Certainely to Heaven 'tis gone
>   The Earth's not worthy of its stay:
>
> For 'tis not possible there should
>   Bee found in all thy glorious Nation
> For such a Spiritt, an equall Mould;
>   ffor, none by Samian=Transmigration
>
> Her Spiritt in herritt could, except shee bee,
>   Some glorious and Immortall Dietie./
>
> Mæstus hæc posivit. Jff[18]

[18] John Parkinson, *Theatrum Botanicum* (London, 1640), Library of Congress, QK41 .P2 Bitting Coll., copy 2, n.p.

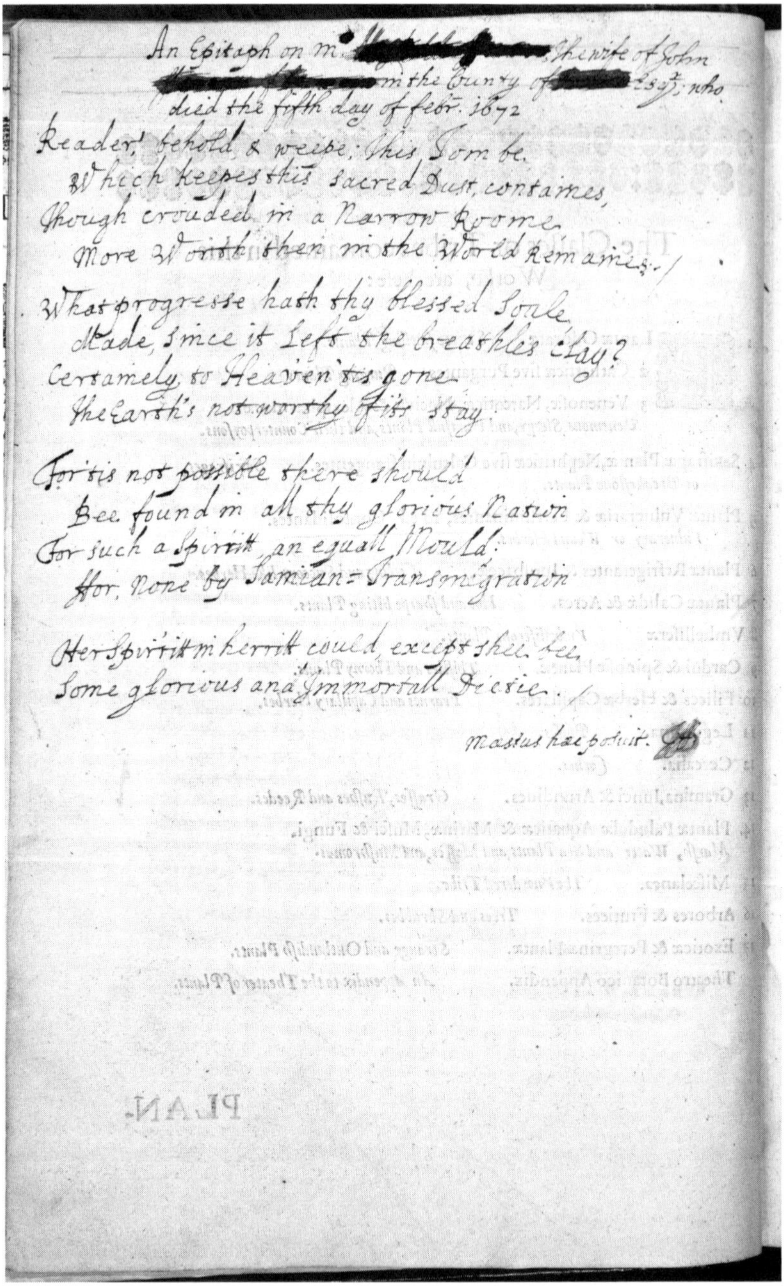

Fig. 2.2 Elegy inscribed by John F. for his wife. John Parkinson's *Theatrum Botanicum*, Library of Congress, QK41 .P2 Bitting Coll., copy 2. Courtesy of the Library of Congress.

Given the eleven-pound bulk of the *Theatrum* (Parkinson's "manlike work of herbs"), there is a certain material logic in making this volume a tombstone upon which is written an epitaph, but another kind of logic emerges when one considers the question of ownership, for this post-Donnean poem has a title, "An Epitaph on M[rs]. [obliterated], the wife of John ff[obliterated] of [obliterated], in the County of D?[obliterated] Esq[r], who died the fifth day of febr[uary]. 1672." This title gives us so much information but withholds key facts at the same time. We have a specific date. We know that this poem was written for a woman who has died. We know her husband's name is John, last name beginning with F. We can almost see a "D" at the beginning of the county name—infrared and high intensity lights in LC conservation give us that much—but an intervening hand armed with a pen and iron gall ink determined that the previous owners' identities and location would be obscured. Yes, a future me wants to waste away in the archives of Devonshire, Derbyshire, Durham, and Dover to find, just maybe, the identity of poet and husband (the Jff at the end would indicate that they are one and the same) and his wife, but for this project, I am more interested in what we can know just from this page[19]—well, and the next—because on the following page, someone has written "M[rs] [Obliterated Obliterated's] Booke" (Figure 2.3). With bright lights, one can make out the initial letters "K" and "F," made more difficult to read still because there seem to be two names, one written on top of another. It is very likely that this is the autograph of the wife grieved for on the previous page. The idea that Mistress F. is an early owner provides another meaning for the poem: the epitaph is written in her book, perhaps her most used book. We begin to wonder about Mistress F. Perhaps she, like Gerard's friend Anne Wilbraham, was a woman particularly known for her skill in medicine. Perhaps, like Catherine Tollemache, she was most remembered in her role as a healer, as that woman was memorialized for her "charity in releeving (through her skill and singular experience in chirugerie) [th]e sick & sore wounded."[20] The extent of the medical knowledge held in the *Theatrum*, the kind of investment it would have been for the family, the husband's choice of where to memorialize his wife, all point to that wife's dedication to the attainment of medical knowledge.

Beyond surmises about John and Mistress F., this signature illustrates for us one very important potential in the inscriptions within a text: an inscription may not only commemorate the current owner's possession but it may also bear witness to the previous owner's passing. A logical reading of dated examples such as "Jane

---

19 My analysis here of "what we can know just from this page" is in part inspired by that performed by Margaret Ezell on other manuscripts during her contributions as visiting faculty to the National Endowment for the Humanities Summer Institute, *The Handwritten Worlds of Early Modern England*, Folger Shakespeare Library, July 25–26, 2005.

20 As quoted by Jeremy Griffiths, "Introduction," *The Tollemache Book of Secrets: A Descriptive Index and Complete Facsimile with an Introduction and Transcriptions together with Catherine Tollemache's Receipts of Pastery, Confectionary & c.* , completed by A. S. G. Edwards (London: The Roxburghe Club, 2001), 3 n. 5.

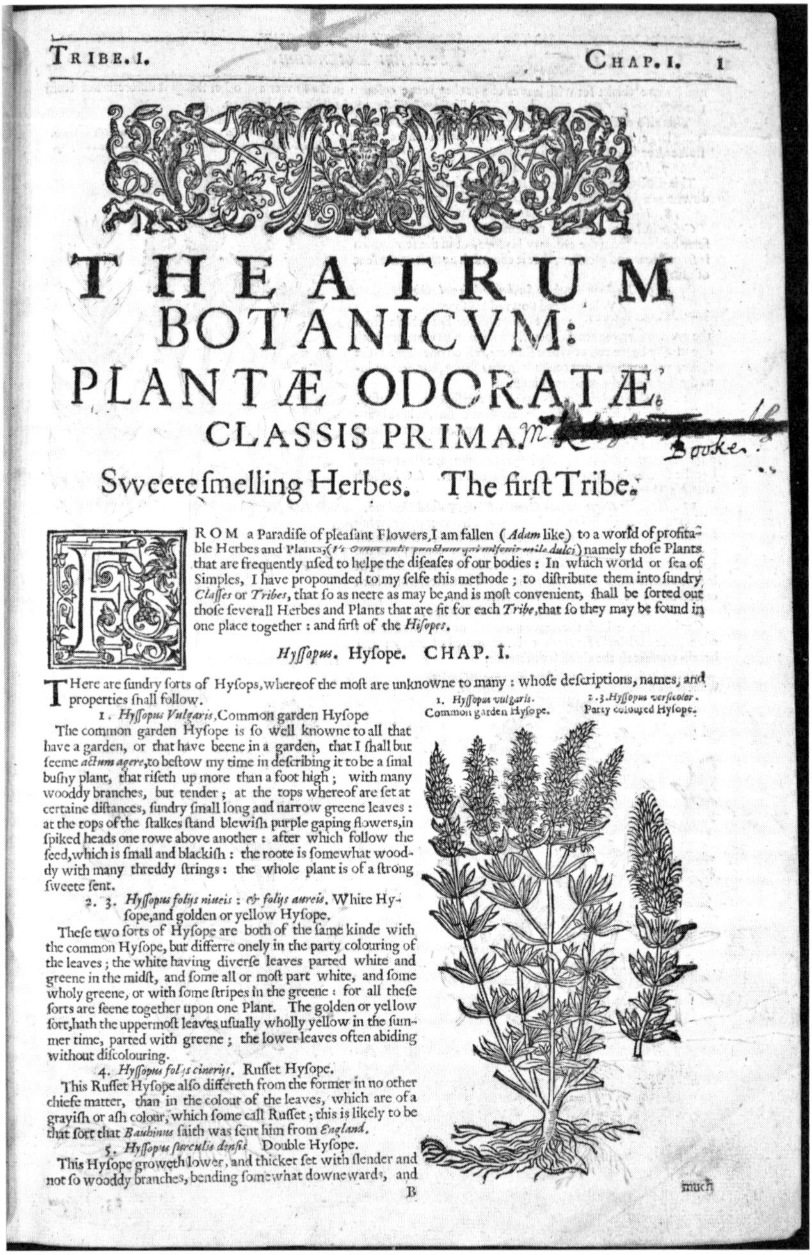
TRIBE. I. CHAP. I. 1

THEATRUM BOTANICVM:

PLANTÆ ODORATÆ

CLASSIS PRIMA. m [redacted] Booke.

Sweete ſmelling Herbes. The firſt Tribe.

FROM a Paradiſe of pleaſant Flowers, I am fallen (*Adam* like) to a world of profitable Herbes and Plants, (*[illegible] dulci*) namely thoſe Plants that are frequently uſed to helpe the diſeaſes of our bodies: In which world or ſea of Simples, I have propounded to my ſelfe this methode; to diſtribute them into ſundry *Claſſes* or *Tribes*, that ſo as neere as may be, and is moſt convenient, ſhall be ſorted out thoſe ſeverall Herbes and Plants that are fit for each *Tribe*, that ſo they may be found in one place together: and firſt of the *Hiſopes*.

Hyſſopus. Hyſope. CHAP. I.

THere are ſundry ſorts of Hyſops, whereof the moſt are unknowne to many: whoſe deſcriptions, names, and properties ſhall follow.

1. *Hyſſopus Vulgaris*, Common garden Hyſope

The common garden Hyſope is ſo well knowne to all that have a garden, or that have beene in a garden, that I ſhall but ſeeme *actum agere*, to beſtow my time in deſcribing it to be a ſmal buſhy plant, that riſeth up more than a foot high; with many wooddy branches, but tender; at the tops whereof are ſet at certaine diſtances, ſundry ſmall long and narrow greene leaves: at the tops of the ſtalkes ſtand blewiſh purple gaping flowers, in ſpiked heads one rowe above another: after which follow the ſeed, which is ſmall and blackiſh: the roote is ſomewhat wooddy with many threddy ſtrings: the whole plant is of a ſtrong ſweete ſent.

2. 3. *Hyſſopus foliis niveis: & foliis aureis.* White Hyſope, and golden or yellow Hyſope.

Theſe two ſorts of Hyſope are both of the ſame kinde with the common Hyſope, but differre onely in the party colouring of the leaves; the white having diverſe leaves parted white and greene in the midſt, and ſome all or moſt part white, and ſome wholy greene, or with ſome ſtripes in the greene: for all theſe ſorts are ſeene together upon one Plant. The golden or yellow ſort, hath the uppermoſt leaves uſually wholly yellow in the ſummer time, parted with greene; the lower leaves often abiding without diſcolouring.

4. *Hyſſopus foliis cineriis.* Ruſſet Hyſope.

This Ruſſet Hyſope alſo differeth from the former in no other chiefe matter, than in the colour of the leaves, which are of a grayiſh or aſh colour, which ſome call Ruſſet; this is likely to be that ſort that *Bauhinus* ſaith was ſent him from *England*.

5. *Hyſſopus ſurculis denſis* Double Hyſope.

This Hyſope groweth lower, and thicker ſet with ſlender and not ſo wooddy branches, bending ſomewhat downewards, and

1. *Hyſſopus vulgaris.* Common garden Hyſope.

2. 3. *Hyſſopus verſicolor.* Party coloured Hyſope.

B much

Fig. 2.3 Woman's obliterated signature, very likely the wife of John F. Library of Congress, QK41 .P2 Bitting Coll., copy 2. Courtesy of the Library of Congress.

Baker 1660" in a *Theatrum Botanicum* at Philadelphia's Academy of Natural Sciences is that the autographer records the date of when she came into possession of the book.[21] The epitaph suggests that an inscription, when juxtaposed to another, may also record the death of a previous owner. Certainly the pairing of John and Mistress F.'s signatures constitutes an overt example, but others may similarly carry a sense of loss or generational transition. If, as Brayman Hackel points out, the "transmission of the volume" is in part "marked" when "the later owners delete the earlier signatures,"[22] might the non-deletion of a previous signature possibly memorialize the previous owner?[23] For example, one copy of John Parkinson's *Paradisi in Sole Paradisus Terrestris* at Texas A&M's Cushing Library contains two signatures with dates on the verso of the dedication to Queen Henrietta Maria. The first, "Sr John Weld Senio^r^ 1666," with its "spiralling flourishes" underneath,[24] literally takes up the entire page (Figure 2.4).[25] Underneath Sir John's name in the first curl of the first flourish, Mary Saltonstall has signed hers with the date 1674. Indeed, the *Alumni Oxonienses* lists a Sir John Welde who died July 11, 1674, so the date that marks the herbal coming into Mary Saltonstall's possession may also mark the passing of Sir John.[26]

Another example related to this question of the death and memorializing of a previous owner is found in the Blocker Collection at the University of Texas Medical Branch.[27] The Blocker 1633 Gerard has evidence of at least three early modern ownerships, two women's and one man's, plus one name penned on the title page that, like Mistress and John F., has been obliterated. On the page containing the Latin dedication to Launcelot Brown is the name "Arthur Stacie" in

---

21 Parkinson, *Theatrum Botanicum*, Academy of Natural Sciences, Philadelphia, QK41 .P23.

22 Another example of such a deletion can be found in the Countway Library of Medicine in Massachusetts. The Reference Librarian, Jack Eckert, has provided me with the following information and a copy of the relevant page from that library's copy of Parkinson's *Theatrum Botanicum*: "The Parkinson . . . has the ownership inscription [crossed out] of Ann Stoughton and, below that, one of Margret Massingberd," e-mail to the author, January 4, 2006. Ann Stoughton's roman hand, still legible despite the crossings, appears to be early modern, Countway Medicine, Rare Books f 1.Me.1.

23 Brayman Hackel, *Reading Material*, 219.

24 Peter Beal, "Feathery Scribe (*fl. c.*1625–1640)," *DNB*, http://www.oxforddnb.com/view/article/75559 (accessed April 27, 2007).

25 John Parkinson, *Paradisi in Sole Paradisus Terrestris* (London, 1629), Texas A&M, Cushing Memorial Library & Archives, Rare Books SB97.P24 1629.

26 University of Oxford, *Alumni Oxonienses*, vol. 1, 1500–1714 (Nendeln/Liechtenstein: Kraus, 1968), 1594.

27 John Gerard, *The Herball or Generall Historie of Plantes, Gathered by Iohn Gerard of London Master in Chirurgerie, Very Much Enlarged and Amended by Thomas Iohnson, Citizen and Apothecarye* (London, 1633), Moody Library, University of Texas Medical Branch, Rare Book Room 4TO.

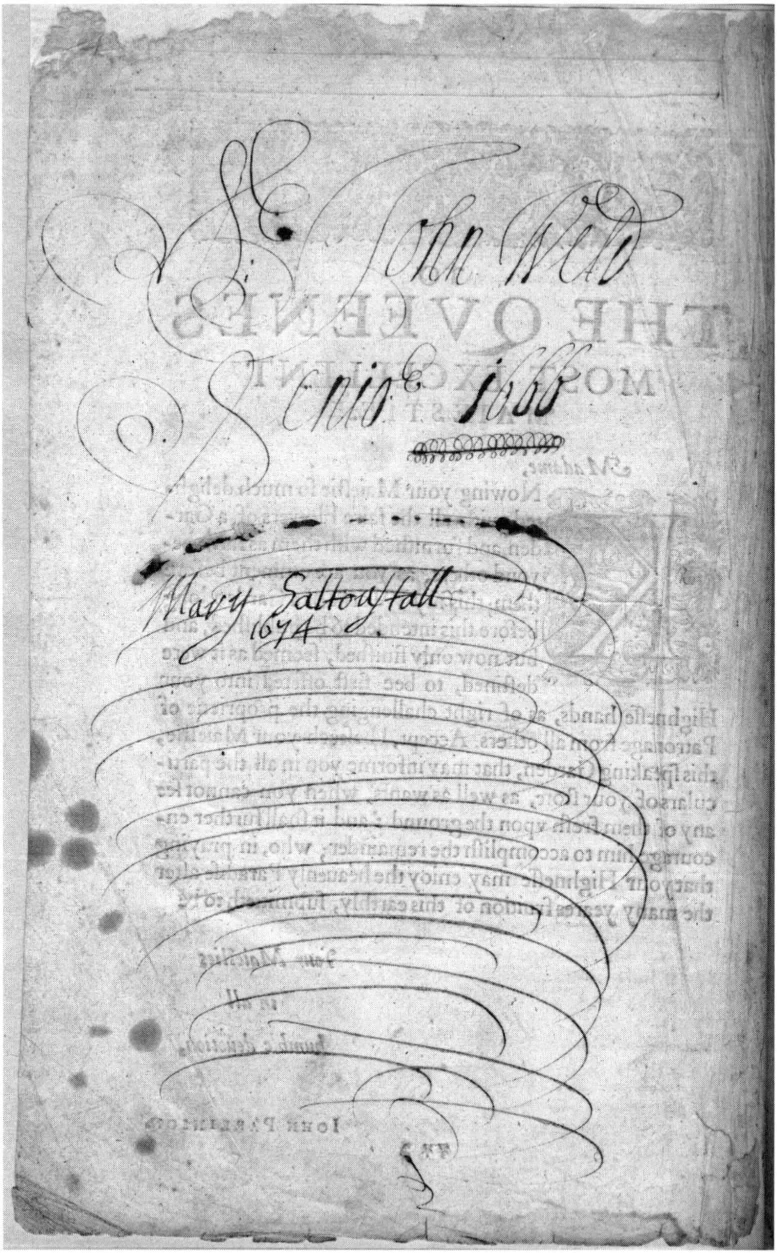

Fig. 2.4 Two related inscriptions from the verso of the dedication. John Parkinson's *Paradisus Terrestris* (1629), Texas A&M, Cushing Library SB97.P24 1629. By permission of the Cushing Memorial Library & Archives.

transitional hand. On the last page, above the *Errata*, in a rounder fully italic hand, is the inscription "Mary Ellys's booke bought of Sister Stacy" (Figure 2.5).

Other aspects of this volume seem attributable to either Mary Ellys or Arthur Stacie. At the bottom of the same page as Mary Ellys's inscription, in studied italic with lobed and accented ascenders and descenders, someone has written

> Blessednes farr off beginneth euen from humility ther is no truer happines in this life then yt which begineth euerlasting happinese, and no truer and no truer [*sic*] and surer misery then that which euen begineth euerlasting misery and they that thinke riches ye cause of happines deceiue them selues no lesse then (Figure 2.5, bottom)

Though this passage is evidently showing someone's best penmanship, the distinctive "o" and "f" found in both Ellys's inscription and the passage supports at least a tentative attribution to the same writer. The exact passage, with slightly different spellings and other corrections, appears in the front materials as well. Neither Ellys's inscription nor the passage directly engages the medical content of the herbal, and one can appreciate the significance of this fact when considering the additions made by Arthur Stacie to the volume.

On the same page as one calligraphic passage, the page bearing the Latin dedication by Thomas Johnson to Richard Edwards, is an element I have not seen in any other herbal, though its inclusion is wonderfully appropriate in such a book (Figure 2.6). In the space above Ellys's passage and below the dedication, someone, a different someone, has drawn a small map of an herb garden, presumably her or his own. With a geometrical design in the center, it has a foursquare layout, with various herbs such as "time," "taragon," and "sorrell" written in each corner. On the south, west, north, and east borders respectively, the artist has placed "Sage," "lavender," "bane," and "hisop" (exchanging the last two in revision). On the other side of a vertical line from the hyssop, written vertically, is "red & damaske roses," a sketch of a hedge or path, "red & damaske," a vertical squiggle, and the word "rosemary." A comparison of Arthur's signature and other notes by him—including a recipe for "a dyet drinke for the dropsie" mostly obscured by repair work—with the writing in the garden makes attribution of the garden to Arthur quite definitive. Moreover, two autographs of the same Arthur Stacie in a book at the Folger Shakespeare Library, "a treatise on poysons" by William Ramesey from 1661, confirms this attribution.[28] Given these coinciding signatures and his various

[28] William Ramesey, *Thanasima Kai Dēlētēria Tractatus de Venenis, or, A Treatise of Poysons: Their sundry sorts, names, natures and virtues, with their severall symptomes, signes diagnosticks, prognosticks, and antidotes* (London, 1661), Folger, Deck C, Rare Book Stacks, 156–278q. The full signature "Arthur Stacie" appears after the prefatory material on the verso before page 1. On the page that begins the address "To the Judicious and Ingenius Reader," Stacie has signed his name "AStacie," with the A and S entwined. More flourishes indicate a different moment than the herbal signature.

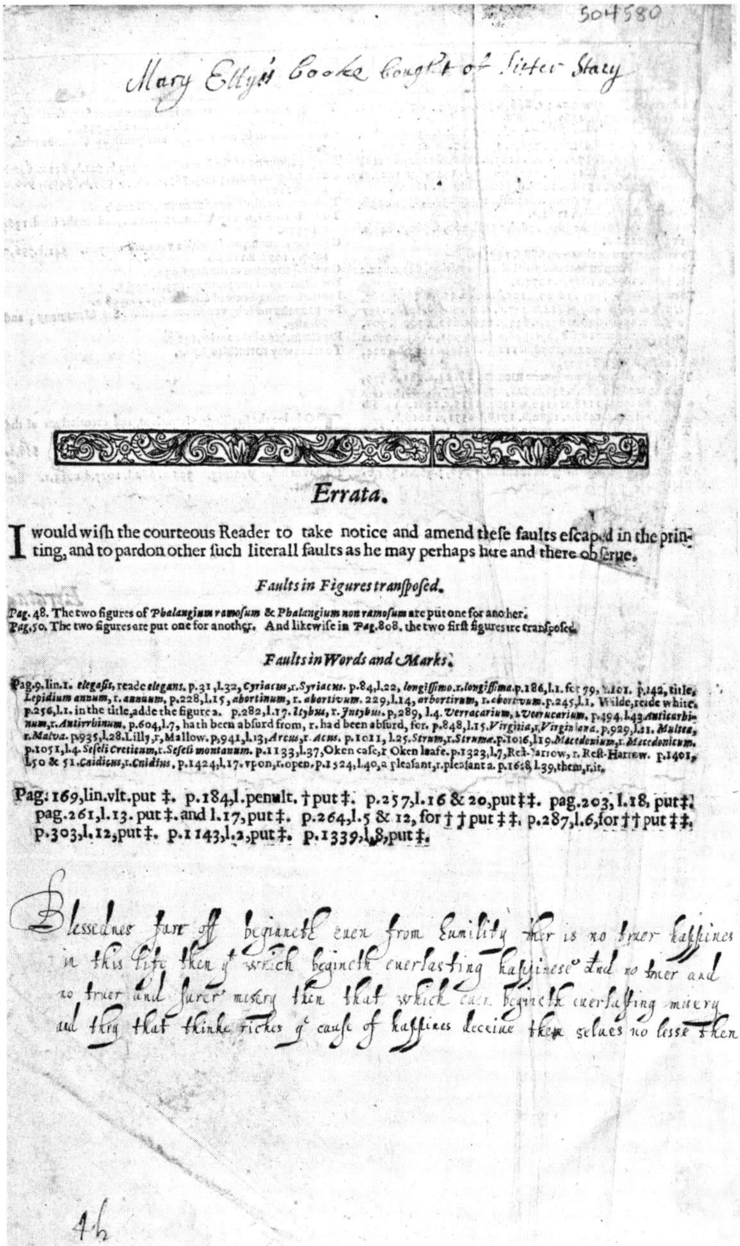

504580

Mary Ellys Booke bought of Sister Stacy

Errata.

I would wiſh the courteous Reader to take notice and amend theſe faults eſcaped in the printing, and to pardon other ſuch literall faults as he may perhaps here and there obſerue.

Faults in Figures tranſpoſed.

Pag. 48. The two figures of *Phalangium ramoſum* & *Phalangium non ramoſum* are put one for another.
Pag. 50. The two figures are put one for another. And likewiſe in Pag. 808. the two firſt figures are tranſpoſed.

Faults in Words and Marks.

Pag. 9. lin. 1. *elegaſis*, reade *elegans*. p. 31, l. 32, *Cyriacus*, r. *Syriacus*. p. 84, l. 22, *longiſſimo*, r. *longiſſima*. p. 186, l. 1. for 79, r. 101. p. 142, title, *Lepidium annum*, r. *annuum*. p. 228, l. 15, *abortinum*, r. *abortivum*. 229, l. 14, *arbortirum*, r. *abortivum*. p. 245, l. 1, Wilde, reade white. p. 256, l. 1. in the title, adde the figure 2. p. 282, l. 17. *Itybus*, r. *Intybus*. p. 289, l. 4. *Verracarium*, r. *Verrucarium*. p. 494, l. 43. *Anticarbinum*, r. *Antirrhinum*. p. 604, l. 7, hath been abſurd from, r. had been abſurd, for. p. 848, l. 15. *Virginia*, r. *Virginiana*. p. 929, l. 21. *Maltea*, r. *Malva*. p. 935, l. 28. Lilly, r. Mallow. p. 941, l. 13, *Arcus*, r. *Acus*. p. 1011, l. 25. *Strum*, r. *Struma*. p. 1016, l. 19. *Macedonium*, r. *Macedonicum*. p. 1051, l. 4. *Seſeli Creticum*, r. *Seſeli montanum*. p. 1133, l. 37, Oken caſe, r. Oken leafe. p. 1323, l. 7, Red-Yarrow, r. Reſt-Harrow. p. 1401, l. 50 & 51. *Cnidicus*, r. *Cnidius*. p. 1424, l. 17. vpon, r. open. p. 1524, l. 40, a pleaſant, r. pleaſant a. p. 1618, l. 39, them, r. it.

Pag. 169, lin. vlt. put ‡. p. 184, l. penult. † put ‡. p. 257, l. 16 & 20, put ‡‡. pag. 203, l. 18, put ‡. pag. 261, l. 13. put ‡. and l. 17, put ‡. p. 264, l. 5 & 12, for †† put ‡‡. p. 287, l. 6, for †† put ‡‡. p. 303, l. 12, put ‡. p. 1143, l. 2, put ‡. p. 1339, l. 8, put ‡.

Blessednes farr off beginneth even from humility ther is no truer happines in this life then yt which beginneth everlasting happinese and no truer and no truer and surer misery then that which ever beginneth everlasting misery and they that thinke riches ye cause of happines deceive them selues no lesse then

46

Fig. 2.5 Inscription on last page that implies two female owners. John Gerard's *Herball* (1633), Moody Library at the University of Texas Medical Branch, Rare Book Room 4TO. By permission of the Moody Library.

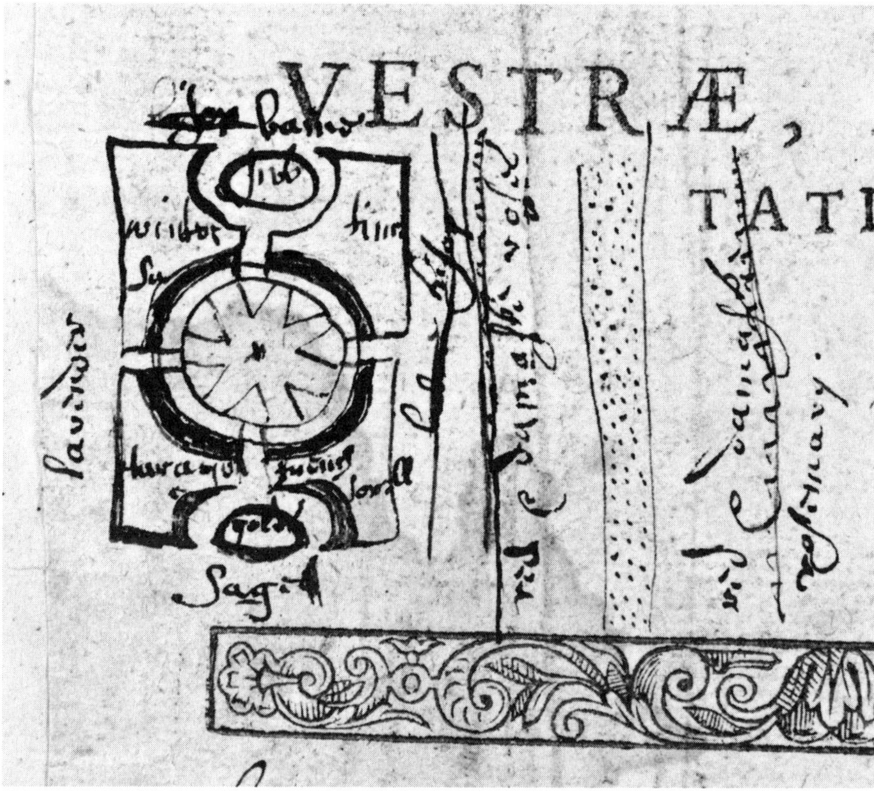

Fig. 2.6 Sketch of garden by Arthur Stacie on the page of the Latin dedicatory letter by Thomas Johnson to Richard Edwards, n.p., 1633 Gerard, Moody Library, UTMB, Rare Book Room 4TO. By permission of the Moody Library.

additions to the herbal, it is clear that Arthur Stacie was the medical practitioner in the Stacie/y household.

Realizing the active presence of Arthur Stacie throughout the volume makes his absence from the inscription "Mary Ellys's booke bought of Sister Stacy" all the more poignant. The early markers in Mary Ellys's writing place hers within proximity to Arthur Stacie's evidently seventeenth-century hand. "Sister Stacy," likely the wife who inherited the book, becomes an intermediary between the presumably dead Arthur and the living and, perhaps, wealthy Ellys. Indeed, the monetary transaction here denotes a certain kind of relationship between the individuals, while the word "Sister" brings with it the possibility that Mary Ellys was the sister of Arthur, "Sister Stacy" being her sister-in-law. Indeed, one of the few christening records of an "Arthur Stacye" in the period exists in Bythorn, Huntingdonshire in 1665, born to parents John and Elizabeth, who seven years previously christened a daughter Mary.[29] Regardless of any determined relationship between the owners, Mary Ellys's purchase of the book marks the end of Arthur Stacie's engaged and engaging relationship to it.

Thus the example of John and Mistress F. demonstrates how a signature left within an authoritative medical text may serve to remind future readers of the medical authority of the book's original owner. Someone who purchases such a large and expensive text that held the medical knowledge of all known plants such as the *Theatrum* or the "enlarged" 1633 Gerard makes a particular kind of investment, presumably not out of casual interest. The preserved inscription in the herbal text can act as a kind of memorial to the deceased individual's medical authority. Not only does the original owner make a claim to that knowledge in signing his or her signature; the next owner also underlines that claim in preserving the first owner's name.

Authority in Place

Another possible relationship between first and subsequent owners is realized through an example found in the 1636 Gerard at Texas A&M's Cushing Library and Archives (Figure 2.7). Written in three separate italic hands on the front flyleaf's recto is the following provenance:[30]

> Sarah Gibson
>
> Gave this Book to
Madam Legge
Madam Legge
Bequeathed it
to Madam Burton
Madam Burton
Bequeathed it to
George Burton
George Burton
gave it out of Good
will to me and
it is now in the
Possession of Ann
Burton but Ann
Burton out of her

---

[29] *Family Search*, http://www.familysearch.org/eng/search/frameset_search.asp (accessed May 1, 2007). I have also considered the possibility that Mary Ellys and the female Stacy belonged to the same religious community, but these christening records make the familial connection the more likely (though not exclusive) reading.

[30] Some of the following discussion has appeared in Rebecca Laroche, "The Burton Herbal," *Notes and Queries* 252.4 (December 2007): 393–95.

Great Bounty hath
allowed it to the use
of the House—But upon
Demand maybe claimed
by me Ann Burton
witness George Burton Junr

Rob[ert] H Selby Hele
rec[eiv]ed it from the
Library of Philip Burton Esqr
given to him by his Daughter
F.E. Horne after her
F^{r} P Burtons decease

The autograph "Sarah Gibson" (Hand A) also appears on the first recto after the title page along with a nineteenth-century signature and at the beginning of "A supplement or Appendix vnto the generall Table" at the back of the book. Most of the inscription, from "Gave this Book" to "George Burton Junr," is in Hand B (which also writes in pencil a recipe "For a sore throat" faintly legible after the inscription) and presumably belongs to the "me" of the twelfth and twenty-first lines. Hand C, a decidedly later hand, presumably belongs to Robert H. Selby Hele.

From this inscription we can identify seven definitive owners and two intermediary figures. Sarah Gibson's signature indicates that she first owned the book before giving it to Madam Legge, who also writes her name ("Madame Legg"), with a very large initial "M" and a secretary "e" in her surname on the verso of the last leaf. While the identities of both Gibson and Legge remain to be determined, the choice of wording—"gave" over "bequeathed"—implies that Gibson was still living when the transfer occurred. The next four owners, in the shared surname of Burton, illustrate familial inheritance, and it is through these family relationships that we can identify key players in this inscription. Madam Burton to George Burton to Ann Burton to Philip Burton is the line of inheritance between Madam Legge and Robert Selby Hele, and the intermediary figures of George Burton, Jr. and F. E. Horne provide any missing links along the way. Historical inquiry soon reveals that Ann Reeve and George Burton, Jr. (c. 1717–1791), noted English clergyman and biblical scholar, were married July 9, 1743.[31] Both husband and wife could be candidates for the writer of the provenance, but given the proximity of "me" and "Ann Burton" in the penultimate line, Ann seems to be the author. Philip Burton, whose daughter Felicia Horne gave the herbal to Selby Hele, survived by one year his younger brother and his wife Felicia, both of

[31] Thompson Cooper, "Burton, George (*bap*. 1717, *d*. 1791)," rev. Emma Major, *DNB* http://www.oxforddnb.com/view/article/4128 (accessed February 21, 2007).

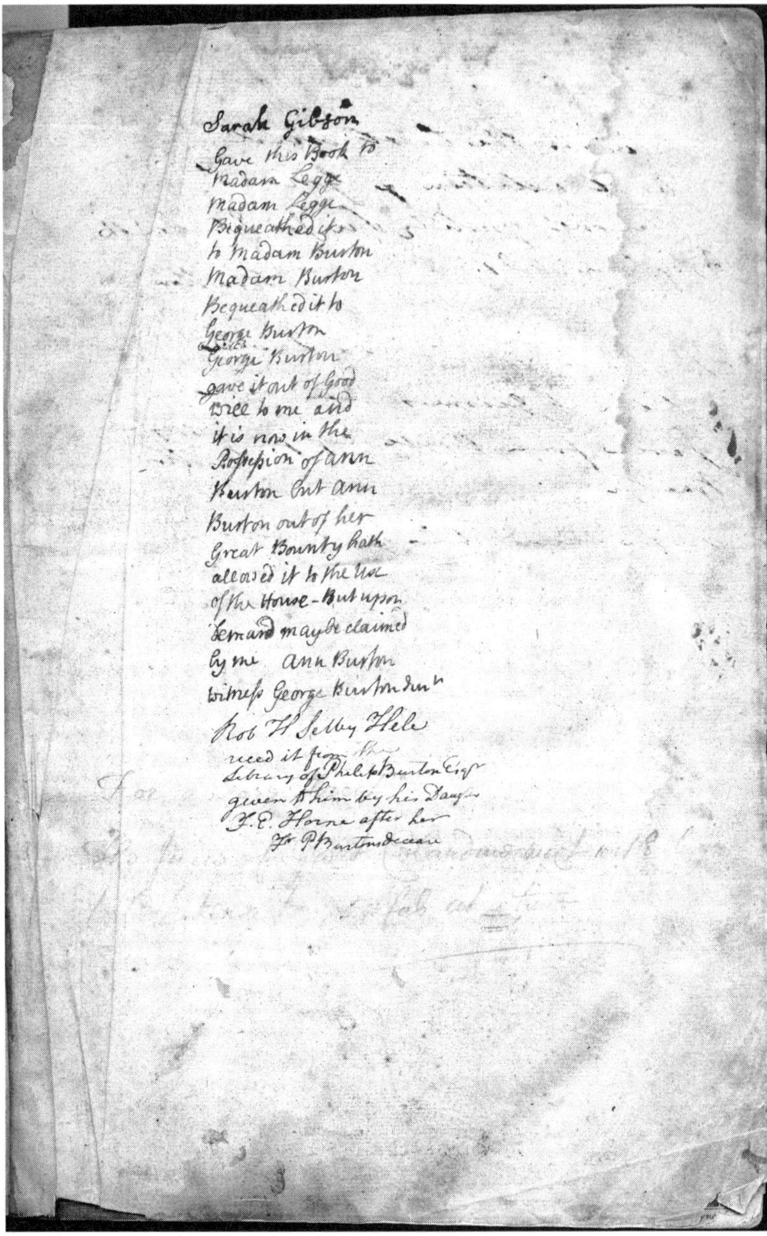

Sarah Gibson
Gave this Book to
Madam Legge
Madam Legge
Bequeathed it
to Madam Burton
Madam Burton
Bequeathed it to
George Burton
George Burton
gave it out of Good
Will to me and
it is now in the
Possession of Ann
Burton But Ann
Burton out of her
Great Bounty hath
allowed it to the use
of the House - But upon
demand may be claimed
by me Ann Burton
witness George Burton Jun
Rob H Selby Hele
recd it from the
Library of Philip Burton Esqr
given him by his Daughter
F. E. Horne after her
Fr P Burtons decease

Fig. 2.7 Provenance in three hands naming seven owners. 1636 Gerard's *Herball*, front flyleaf recto, Texas A&M Cushing Library, QK41 .G3 1636. By permission of the Cushing Memorial Library & Archives.

whom died in 1791.[32] The George Burton who "gave it out of Good will to me" ostensibly could be Ann's husband, but the omission of the "Junr" from the name when it is included in the witness line below indicates that the man in question is likely Ann's father-in-law. As Ann does not provide Madam Burton's first name, we can only make assumptions about her identity, but whatever her relationship to George Burton, Senior—mother, wife (née Elizabeth Denton), or aunt—she predeceases him.

Finding such a ownership history with notable owners is certainly a marvelous occurrence in and of itself,[33] but this particular inscription may also give us further insight into the occasion that prompts such writing. Ann Burton authors the history at a particular moment, the "now" of the thirteenth line. The giving of the book to Ann may have been prompted by either Ann and George's wedding or the death of Madam Burton, and with the book came its oral history, but the writing of that history in the inscription comes at a different instigation, perhaps contemporary with receiving the book, the lending of the book to "the House," thus marking the text "return to lender." That Ann Burton writes "the House," rather than "her House," reflects the fact that during their marriage George was rector of Eldon, then of Herringswell, both in Suffolk.[34] "The House" thus refers to the great house to which the rectory would have been attached. In this light, the writing of the provenance emphasizes the necessity of the book's return: even though it may be of more use in the larger house, the herbal must come back to the rightful owners because it is a book with family history. That it was so rightfully returned is evidenced in its position in Philip Burton's library upon his death, as Ann and George had no children.

The context provided within the ownership history for the writing of that history thus distinguishes it from similar inscriptions. This is not simply a genealogy found in so many Bibles and books of hours as discussed by William Sherman and Mary Erler.[35] Presumably such devotional texts would have a stationary place within the home and would not be lent out to neighbors. What is more, it provides a history of the book over a history of the family; the absence of dates and Madam Burton's Christian name means that the family history is incomplete. Thus this inscription written against the loan could be a version of other related motivations; that is, in signing his or her name, an individual might be attempting to protect the

---

[32] Daniel Lysons, "Eltham," *The Environs of London: Volume 4: Counties of Herts, Essex & Kent* (1796), 394–421, http://www.british-history.ac.uk/report.asp?compid=45484 (accessed March 29, 2007), 6.

[33] Brayman Hackel calls analagous rare examples "delicious," *Reading Material*, 219. I have to agree.

[34] Cooper, "Burton, George."

[35] Sherman, *Used Books*, 59–60; Erler, *Women, Reading, and Piety*, 119. This practice is partly seen in the University of Pennsylvania *A Nievve Herball* (1578), where someone has listed the children of Joseph and Susannah Barker next to the portrait of Dodoens, RBC Folio 580 D665 EL.

book in question from being subsumed into a larger library, as Brayman Hackel and Morgan have argued.[36] Writing from within the larger group, the inscriber designates her or himself the person to whom the book ultimately belongs.

Unlike the intervening owners of the *Theatrum Botanicum* discussed in the previous section, Burton does not obliterate or memorialize previous owners for their own sake, but rather she preserves the book's history for the articulation of the book's personal as well as material value. Most immediately, Ann Burton's inscription allows us to give an approximate date to Sarah Gibson's signature: if the "now" signifies a date in or around 1743, then this could easily place Gibson somewhere in the late seventeenth or early eighteenth century.[37] In registering her ownership along with those before her in the book, Ann Burton distinguishes the herbal from other holdings in what one imagines to be a large household, and it is this insight that illuminates other examples of herbal inscriptions. In the broader context of women's ownership of herbals, this provenance thus has profound implications for the articulation of women's libraries.

This analysis might remind us of that concerning Frances Wolfreston. Morgan has argued that Frances's signatures in her extensive library in part served to distinguish her collection from that of her son, who also had "antiquarian tastes."[38] Along with denoting ownership and everything that goes with it, the inscription may also signify its position in the house, saying "if found return to Mistress X's chambers."[39] Such instances recall the medical reading and experimentation that sometimes occurred in women's closets outlined by Lena Cowen Orlin's cultural survey, suggesting an even more specific place designated by the signature.[40] Within the record of herbal ownership, we have instances of Elizabeth Freke, who catalogs the "abstractt of Gerralds herball of my wrightine" among her books in her closet,[41] and Elizabeth Isham, whose closet held a vial filled with swallowwort oil made by her great-grandmother. In this way, a woman's books may be hers in where they are kept—i.e., on certain shelves or in a trunk within a woman's

36 See note 15 above.

37 Another supporting piece of evidence for this dating can be found on the verso of the flyleaf, where beside a nineteenth-century description of the book are two neatly written dates, the first below the other, "1636" and "1720," in what looks to be hand D. If 1720 is the date of ownership, the juxtaposition meaning to calculate the age of the book, then, as the hand does not belong to Gibson or Legge, the notation may belong to either Madam or George Burton, the third or fourth owner.

38 Morgan, "Frances Wolfreston," 201.

39 Brayman Hackel makes a similar point in *Reading Material*, 215. See also Laroche, "Catherine Tollemache's Library."

40 Lena Cowen Orlin, "Gertrude's Closet," *Shakespeare Jahrbuch* 134 (1998): 44–67.

41 Elizabeth Freke, *The Remembrances of Elizabeth Freke, 1671–1714*, ed. Raymond Anselment (Cambridge: Cambridge University Press for the Royal Historical Society, 2001), 175.

closet—and her books, always bearing her name, may rotate in and out of the larger household.[42]

The idea that the signature designates not only the book's owner but also its position in the household may be further developed through the inscription "Katherine Shirley her booke" found in the *Paradisus Terrestris* in the Arizona State University Patten Collection.[43] In addition to the inscription, the bookplate of Washington Sewallis, Earl Ferrers from 1842 to 1859, and the impresa of the Shirley arms on the calf binding give nearly conclusive evidence that the woman behind the signature was Katherine Okeover Shirley (d. 1672), wife (m. 1646) to Robert, fourth baronet (1629–1656), and mother to Robert, first Earl Ferrers (1650–1717).[44] Without a corresponding signature, it is difficult to be one hundred percent certain, but the two other pieces of evidence locate the book in the Ferrers collection, either at Staunton Harold or at Tamworth Castle, as late as the nineteenth century, which would put the book somewhere in the Ferrers line of descent. The only other "Katherine" in the direct line is Catherine Cotton Shirley, (1733–1786), wife of the sixth Earl Ferrers, who lived quite late for the variant spellings and for the purchase of a book printed in 1629. This analysis assumes that other Katherines born into the Shirley line, such as Robert and Katherine's eldest daughter, Katherine Shirley Venables, would have taken a book that they had designated their own out of the house with them when they married as part of their dowry. In such an assumption, I anticipate the example discussed below of Grace Mildmay, who seems to bring her girlhood edition of Turner with her when she moves in with her in-laws.

The constellation of evidence in this particular volume locates it not only historically but also geographically. Its identification with the Ferrers library locates it within a certain house, as well as with a certain person. If correct, the identification of "Katherine Shirley" as the wife of the royalist Sir Robert Shirley tells us that she left the volume behind when she moved from that estate after her husband's death from suspicious circumstances in the Tower of London in 1656 and that it was not with the property she took with her to Staffordshire and Northamptonshire where she spent her widowhood. In her probate will, she leaves "The best Booke in my Closet, except my gilt Bible with knobs" to Mistress Katherine Dalbin, not of the Ferrers line (we are not so lucky as in the example of Sara Gater to have Shirley name the *Paradisus* as part of her bequest),[45] and the rest of her property, minus two horses and various moneys for servants and the

---

42 Brayman Hackel, *Reading Material*, 214–15.

43 Parkinson, *Paradisus Terrestris*, Hayden Special Collection SPEC, P–138.

44 M. Dorman, "Shirley, Sir Robert, fourth baronet (1629–1656)," *DNB*, http://www.oxforddnb.com/view/article/25434 (accessed January 23, 2007).

45 Evelyn Philip Shirley, *Stemmata Shirleiana; or the Annals of the Shirley Family, Lords of Nether Etindon in the County of Warwick, and of Shirley in the County of Derby* (London: Nichols and Sons, 1873); Katherine Shirley, "Will," Public Records Office, Prob. 11/341, fol. 12v. On the record of Gater's Gerard, see Nagy, *Popular Medicine*, 66.

purchase of commemorative rings by other family members and friends, goes to her "dearest Daughter Dorothy Shirley," who seems to have been with her through her final illness.[46] Thus the inscription of "Katherine Shirley her booke" distinguished the book from others in the family book collection as long as Katherine Shirley resided within Staunton Harold, but once she was removed from that location and her book stayed behind, the signature changed in signification. Once Katherine Shirley had passed on, the book now was marked with familial provenance and thus belonged to Staunton Harold and with it to the Shirley inheritance. We see this turn in signification when Sarah Gibson's and Madam Legge's inscriptions, originally meant to denote their ownership, are then appropriated by Ann Burton in denoting the book's history and thus its value.

Through the example of the Burton herbal, we may thus come to read inscriptions from two different vantages. In the relationship between smaller book collections and larger ones, inscriptions such as "Katherine Shirley her booke"—and with them perhaps "M^{rs} K[obliterated] F[obliterated's] Booke," "Anne Whitehall of Yildersley her booke 1672," "Anne Purefey her booke," and "Ann Loggin her boock" gain inflection.[47] That is, if the signatures were in part meant to distinguish a woman's books within the larger family library, might the immediate intended audience read the signatures with added emphasis on the first name: "*Katherine* Shirley her booke," "*Anne* Whitehall of Yildersley her booke," "*Anne* Purefey her booke," "*Ann* Loggin her boock"? With her inscription, the woman locates the book in her library against those books belonging to the rest of the household.

In the sense that later signatures cause a change in the original signification, however, we may find sometimes a double inflection. In the case of Anne Whitehall, for example, the current owner writes her name against two previous owners, a Charles Whitehall, whose Latin inscription is dated 1651, and another Anne Whitehall, who writes "Ann Whithall is the owner of this booke" in an earlier, less assured roman hand.[48] Therefore, we may read the italic and English inscription as "*Anne* Whitehall *of Yildersley* her booke 1672," making it not only a version of the inscription, "Elizabeth Hunt her Book *not* his," shared by Brayman Hackel, but also a version of "her book *not hers*."[49] Anne of Yildersley does not cross out the previous owners because they are her family, thus memorializing them and retaining family history and importance; nonetheless she asserts an authority that is separate from those of preceding generations. The woman thus

---

46 K. Shirley, "Will," fol. 12v.

47 The last of these is found in Parkinson, *Theatrum Botanicum*, Library of Congress, QK41 .P2 English Print Folio, copy 1.

48 Dodoens, *A Nievve Herball* (1578), University of Pennsylvania, RBC Folio 580 D665 EL. Charles's Latin inscription appears on page 465, at the end of the third book and his initials appear on the title page. Ann Whitehall's claim to ownership appears on the verso of the title page. She also experiments with her signature twice at the end of the Latin dedication by Thomas Newton.

49 Brayman Hackel, *Reading Material*, 215.

claims ownership of the herbal text and all the knowledge it contains against and in line with not only those owning other books in the house but also against those who had previously owned the book itself.

The example of the Burton herbal demonstrates several aspects of herbal ownership that we may take into the rest of our discussion. When the individual abdicates ownership, she gives the herbal not only to another person but also to "the house." It is against and within that original context of family and place that the signature gains signification. In the individual's lifetime, the woman claims herbal knowledge and the book's place within her own collection. After her lifetime, as a book with personal and familial history, the expensive volume gains another kind of value, again only within a particular library and as long as it belongs to a particular setting within a particular house. When the individual gives up ownership, she not only gives it to another person, she gives it up to "the house." Thus in signing one's name, one is locating medical authority within one's closet within one's house, and when one abdicates the book, one may also give up the authority found in the book, the position that comes with that authority, and the literal place to which it belongs.

Authority in Status

Another inscription within a volume that is part herbal, part gardening manual, part picture-book challenges our assumptions about the use of medical texts at the same time as it raises questions about the sharing of knowledge between women of different status. A volume of Parkinson's *Paradisus Terrestris* at the Folger has the following inscription on its title page "Anne Purefey [Purefoy] her booke giuen her by her deare sister the Lady ffranklyn June 22th 1643."[50] While Jane Donawerth may see in this an example of the gift exchange of herbal medicine between women,[51] Linda Levy Peck finds evidence in it for her analysis of the leisured origins of luxury.[52] As discussed in Chapter 1, Parkinson's text itself

---

50 I am grateful to Linda Levy Peck for drawing my attention to this inscription. Parkinson, *Paradisus Terrestris*, Folger STC 19300 Copy 1. Some of this analysis appears in Laroche, "To take in hand the practise of physick."

51 Jane Donawerth, "Women's Poetry and the Tudor–Stuart System of Gift Exchange," in *Women, Writing, and the Reproduction of Culture in Tudor and Stuart Britain*, ed. Mary E. Burke, Jane Donawerth, Linda L. Dove, and Karen Nelson, (New York: Syracuse University Press, 2000), 14. A lengthy discussion of recipe exchanges can also be found in Elaine Leong and Sara Pennell, "Recipe Collections and Medical Knowledge," *Medicine and the Market in England and Its Colonies, c. 1450–c. 1850*, ed. Mark S. R. Jenner and Patrick Wallis (Basingstoke, Hampshire: Palgrave Macmillan, 2007), 137–43.

52 Linda Levy Peck, *Consuming Splendor: Society and Culture in Seventeenth-Century England* (Cambridge: Cambridge University Press, 2005), 226. Deborah Harkness repeatedly refers to "ladies" who "bought up copies [of Gerard's herbal] so that they could

distinguishes between "the knowledge . . . [of] what Herbes and Fruits were fit, eyther for Meate or Medicine, for Vse or for Delight," and the text is divided into sections called "The Garden of Pleasure" and "The Kitchen Garden." Even in this division, however, he describes many plants in both sections that have both "use" and "delight" aspects to them.[53] In the end, the text itself begs the question of whether it is a volume indicative of women's medicine or one of women's leisure.

The pages of the Folger *Paradisus*, as Peck points out, show the dalliance of occasional painting of illustrations, which are large and undetailed. Are we to assume that this painting was done by the female hand, presumably Purefoy's? In describing as it does the "ordering of the Garden of Pleasure" and the "delights" to be found in flowers, the text would seem to invite such embellishment, especially in the winter months when an actual garden would not be available for the passing of pleasurable hours. Alluding to less verdant times of year, Parkinson presents the *Paradisus* into "the hands" of Queen Henrietta Maria and writes in his dedication to her that "this speaking Garden . . . may informe you in all the particulars of your store, as well as wants, when you cannot see them fresh vpon the ground" (sig. **2r). In light of the author's prefatory materials, the woman's hand in the Folger volume is one of dalliance and thus subscribes to the women's role as described in its opening pages.

Again, as the gender analysis in Chapter 1 has demonstrated, however, a central tension in the *Paradisus Terrestris* comes from the ways in which this text specifically, but also the print herbal tradition in general (into which Eleanour Rohde places the *Paradisus* while admitting it is "strictly not a herbal, but a gardening book"),[54] facilitates the practice of medicine by women at the same time that it increasingly circumscribes it with a concept of "feminine" endeavors. As the most feminized of the volumes in the early tradition, the *Paradisus* includes various medicinal virtues of plants, while giving equal time to decorative foliage and often highlighting the plants' value in cosmetics. Because of the publicly recognized cultural practice of gentlewomen taking care of the health of their household and their poor neighbors, however, Parkinson includes basic medical information; for example, "All the kindes of Cranes bils are accounted great wound herbes, and effectuall to stay bleedings" (230). If we were to read this text as existing purely

---

trace the illustrations in their embroidery and consult its medical lore," which suggests a possible leisured relationship to all herbals, though the open-leafed quality of illustrations in *Paradisus* seem more suited to the purpose; Deborah Harkness, *The Jewel House: Elizabethan London and the Scientific Revolution* (New Haven: Yale University Press, 2007), 15. For further discussion of the use of herbal texts in embroidery, see the section on Elizabeth Isham in Chapter 3.

53 Parkinson, *Paradisus Terrestris*, sig. **3r; subsequent citations included in text.

54 Eleanour Sinclair Rohde, *The Old English Herbals* (1922; reprint New York: Dover Publications, Inc., 1971), 142. I address the fluid genre of this volume at length in Chapter 1.

for our leisure, then we would need to account for the inclusion of medicinal aspects of the herbs.

The handwritten inscription in the volume may provide a means of furthering our analysis, as it indicates two relationships to its pages: one that relates to it as a female head of household, one as a yet-unmarried girl. We need to consider the possibility that perhaps the two sisters saw the volume differently. Elizabeth Franklin, wife of a Parliament member and mother of seventeen children by the time of his death in 1647, may have valued the volume for its medical and other practical knowledge.[55] Indeed, with her husband's position in London, as we have seen in the example of Elizabeth Bagot at the beginning of this chapter and will see with Grace Mildmay in the next chapter, it is likely Lady Franklin had many duties to oversee, not the least of which was the maintenance of the health of the household.

Anne Purefoy, still in her father George Purefoy's household at the time of the gift, certainly not in charge of any caregiving, perhaps saw a source for embroidery patterns (as will be discussed in Chapter 3 in relation to Elizabeth Isham) and pages for painting. Then again (as we will also see in the case of Isham), who is to say that her purposes for the book did not change over time? While a girl, Anne may have viewed the volume as a source of diversion; she may, however, have seen the *Paradisus* as essential reading in her girlhood education, as herbals were read by the young Anne Clifford (discussed in the introduction) and Grace Mildmay (in Chapter 3), and thus a resource in her future household work. Again, in anticipating our discussion of Elizabeth Isham and the memorializing of family illness, life experience may bring a reader to the medical knowledge included in a book that has proven to be a resource in other aspects of life. A reader's relationship to a text necessarily changes over time.

It is important to realize that not all owners of herbal texts used them in the same way. We need only think of the difference between the calligraphic traces of Mary Ellys versus those more studied additions by Arthur Stacie to find such evidence in our cited examples thus far. This possibility of various uses is perhaps strongest in examples of the *Paradisus*, which, though belonging to the herbal tradition as I have argued, presents many purposes within its pages; one may read it for medical content, gardening procedures, embroidery patterns, or cosmetic tips.[56] The

---

[55] Daniel Lysons, *The Environs of London: Being an Historical Account of the Towns Villages, and Hamlets, within Twelve Miles of That Capital,* vol. 3 (London, 1795), 618. My thanks to Jason Powell for his help in finding this information. Online edition available at *British History Online*, http://www.british-history.ac.uk/report.aspx?compid=45453 (accessed March 10, 2009).

[56] In a moment in the Northamptonshire diary discussed below, Isham says that she learned about the medicinal properties of herbs from "a booke which my Sister borrowed of Gardening," Northamptonshire Records Office, IL 3365. My discussion in Chapter 3 posits that the book in question is Parkinson's *Paradisus*. Also, though outside of the date limits, an early modern inscription on the title page of the 1656 *Paradisus* in the Harry Ransom

Purefoy example prompts us to observe the various relationships women may have to medicinal plants and recognizes that when a specific early modern woman uses a botanical trope or refers to picking flowers, she places herself in the continuum between one who enjoys flowers as purely decorative and one who seeks plants as pure medicine, recognizing of course that, as Parkinson's volume shows us, these two extremes are often intertwined. In between these extremes, one may find the recreational aspects of gardening as discussed by Jennifer Munroe and Rebecca Bushnell and, in later developments analyzed by Ann Shteir, the rigors of scientific inquiry.[57] Those women invoking the medicinal end of the spectrum do give us certain markers. Not only do they describe plants as "wholesome" or "healthful," they give the plants a context that emphasizes their medicinal worth. Among the herbal inscriptions themselves, Mary Chambers and Ann Burton both write recipes (as well as Arthur Stacie) on the blank pages of their volumes, indicating the medical practice that accompanies their herbal reading.[58] In other writings, when Lady Margaret Hoby records in her diary that she and her women have gone for a walk into the fields, the context provided by the diary of her religious nonconformity and steady practice in physic indicates that they were not picking bouquets to adorn the house but were more likely looking for medicinal herbs. As another example still, when Brilliana Harley includes a piece of angelica root with a letter to her son in London, it is not for his studies in botany, but explicitly for him to "bite sometimes of" as a preventative against the plague that threatens the city.[59] With some of the inscriptions in this chapter, it is difficult to determine how the text was used, but the particular text purchased—e.g., the *Theatrum* over the *Paradisus*—can give us stronger indications. If we read Anne Purefoy's hand in a volume as only dabbling in the herbal tradition, we see her thus replicating the "dainty delight" prescribed for her in its pages, but if we read against these authorial prescriptions and recognize the presence of her sister, a female head of a large household, we may read other ways in which the volume functioned. The

---

Center Book Collection says that the book provides the "names of every Flower and Shrubb and the nature of them in the use of Phisick," Q SB97 P247p 1656, thus indicating a contemporary emphasis on the medical aspects of the "gardening book."

57 Ann B. Shteir recognizes that, before 1650, women "worked with plants in the herbal tradition of home-based medical practices," *Cultivating Women, Cultivating Science* (Baltimore: Johns Hopkins University Press, 1996), 4. Jennifer Munroe, "Inheritance, Land, and the Garden Space for Women in Aemilia Lanyer's *Salve Deus Rex Judaeorum*," *Gender and the Garden in Early Modern English Literature* (Burlington, Vermont: Ashgate Publishing, 2008), 75–96; Rebecca Bushnell, *Green Desire: Imagining Early Modern English Gardens* (Ithaca, New York: Cornell University Press, 2007).

58 Mary Chambers writes her recipe on the last flyleaf of *A Nievve Herball*, Linnaean Society Library, RF.578, Another Copy. Ann Burton's recipe appears in pencil underneath the provenance described above.

59 Brilliana Harley, *Letters of the Lady Brilliana Harley*, 129. For comparison see Maria Thynne's letter to her husband that tells him to take "3 or fower leaves of rue" with raisins, transcribed in *Lay by Your Needles Ladies*, 77.

medicinal information in that volume, relatively limited as it may be, thus gains importance. Then again, perhaps the book's attractiveness as a gift was its variety of functions. So while we should never discount the possibility that these texts were used in medical practice, in the end, we can take these prescriptive volumes only for the information they give and cannot presume to know definitively how they were used; we can look only for clues.

Consequently, our third inscription recognizes that medical authority is not a given referent in herbal writing. Unlike the case of Mistress F., whose memorial exists in an herbal text focused on the medicinal aspects of plants, and the "great bounty" of Ann Burton that recognized the value of such a volume to a large household, Anne Purefoy's *Paradisus* is not clearly medicinal in its use. What the Purefoy case prompts in our analysis, however, is the idea that one's relationship to medical authority may change over time as one's social roles permute and new skill sets develop. Thus we must ask for other social signifiers surrounding herbal texts in order to better understand how medical authority may or may not be a part of herbal ownership and, by extension, herbal reading and writing. More pointedly, we must consider the processes of acquiring literacy and pursuing education that inform and change a woman's relationship to established medical authority as she acquires her own.

Authority in Education

Our final example evidences one woman's possible beginnings with herbal knowledge and writing literacy. "Ownership" in this case is less about material possession and more about knowledge acquisition, and this distinction adds further nuance to our understanding of the term. A woman may come into the possession of an herbal without studying it, and another may come to read it in an associate's chambers. In both cases, the woman's relationship to medical authority may shift later in life; that is, the first woman may find reason to begin studying her herbal or the latter may acquire her own text, either through copying or purchase. We will witness this shift through the narration of Elizabeth Isham, but it is here, in the signature of Ann Parsons, that we can see that a woman's name in an herbal registers one moment in a woman's acquisition of herbal knowledge, and the authority with which she signs her name may tell us something about where that moment occurs in a life.

The dominant inscription in the 1619 Dodoens at the New York Public Library is "Sum liber Richard: Parsons: Anno. 1628," written in roman hand on the flyleaf recto just before the title page (Figure 2.8a). Parsons surrounds his signature with "spiralling flourishes,"[60] and other hands have added their scribbles, including some ornate "Rs" and the inscription "By me Jhon Parsons" (with a secretary "e") on the bottom and inverted. The aspect of this volume that most interests us,

[60] Beal, "Feathery Scribe."

however, is another autograph, one found in the table of virtues at the back of the book, on verso 3E3, the name "Ann Parsos" (Figure 2.8b). My analysis begins with the assumption that "Ann Parsons" is the intended signature and that this faulty execution is significant: this is not someone who is comfortable writing her name. When we consider the woman's autograph next to the highly elaborate work of Richard Parsons, an even more exciting realization surfaces: she is imitating the more elaborate signature as a handwriting guide, or Richard Parsons has provided the guide separately. Regardless, the similarities between the "Ann" of those same letters from Richard's "Anno" and the two executions of "Parsons" (the tails of the "As" and "Ps" and the particularities of the letters "n," "r," and "s") makes it clear that Richard's hand is mixed up with Ann's handwriting attempts and that she may be using the herbal as space for practice.[61] The idea that she may also be reading the herbal in her girlhood instruction is supported by the examples of Ann Purefoy and Anne Clifford from above and that of Grace Mildmay discussed below, but in this case, it would be difficult for us to assume material ownership based on the signature. Ann's position in Richard's library is one of a student, leading us to conjecture that this may be an instance of father and daughter imitation or instruction. It does not seem, however, that Ann eventually inherits the herbal; the signature of John Parsons on the title page versus Ann's hidden signature in the index would point to its maintenance in the male line. John's signature claims material ownership of the volume, while Ann's is less assertive.

Ann's obscurity and hesitancy point to an aspect of signatures that bears closer inspection. Richard Parsons's flourishes do not have a counterpart in the women's examples I have uncovered. The nearest I have found are Elizabeth Bagot's marvelous "B," Madam Legge's massive "M," and the final colons without an abbreviating function in both Bagot's signature and Elizabeth Turner's autograph on the verso of the title page in the Huntington Library's 1578 Dodoens.[62] We may consider one aspect of some of these signatures a kind of flourish, however: their position in the book. Elizabeth Bagot, Jane Baker, and Elizabeth Hamond (from the Houghton's 1578 *Nievve Herball*)[63] all put their names on the title page itself, and Elizabeth Turner and Sarah Gibson do so at the top of the next possible page as there seems to be little space on their respective title pages. In this positioning these

---

[61] Ezell has pointed to examples of such imitation in "domestic papers" in NEH Summer Institute *The Handwritten Worlds*. Sherman discusses them in *Used Books*. See also the example discussed by Edith Snook, *Women, Reading, and the Cultural Politics of Early Modern England* (Aldershot, Hampshire: Ashgate Publshing, 2005), 17. Another example of practicing in different hands and languages can be found in the Princeton 1619 Dodoens (Rare Books (EX), Oversize 8707.303q), in which John Baker writes his name in roman and italic hand and in English and in Latin.

[62] Dodoens, *A Nievve Herball* (1578), Huntington Library, Rare Books 60102 (reproduced in the database *Early English Books Online*, http://eebo.chadwyck.com).

[63] Elizabeth Hamond's signature is found in Dodoens's *Nievve Herball* (1578), Houghton Library, f STC 6984.

women denote their ownership with authority. Yes, this is common practice across genders, but to do so as a woman in the period undoes many preconceptions about women's modesty, a motif recurrent in the writings considered in the following chapters.

Another aspect of the Parsons case further illumines some of our other autographs: in writing her name, a woman may also be practicing her signature. We have seen how in Elizabeth Bagot's herbal she attempts one "B" to mark it out and replace it with one better executed. Similarly, Katherine Shirley blots the "i" in "Shirley." In both of these instances, these signatures were likely written in the early years of their marriages when they are getting used to writing a new surname. The idea of practice may also help to explain multiple signatures in one text. Jane Baker signs her name twice on the title page, perhaps to make it more visible at the top when it is otherwise crowded in the middle, but also with a dash of practice in it. Ann Loggin writes her name twice in a Library of Congress *Theatrum*; the early "Ann Whithall" employs her roman signature three times (twice on the same page), and, as we have seen, Sarah Gibson signs her name in three different places in her herbal. In some sense, the owning of the book becomes an occasion for such practice, but it is the position of the signatures and their very repetition that denotes ownership. Ann Parsons's lone signature on a buried page in the index signifies a pen that may not want to be conspicuous and may want to keep its practice hidden. The more often and the more prominently one signs one's name, the more the book belongs to one. Thus the Parsons example allows us to see the difference between a simple signature and a signature that denotes ownership.

Nonetheless, because of her signature, we know that Ann Parsons existed. We also know that she had access to an herbal and that she had occasion to look at, even read, that herbal. We already have evidence in this study of the herbal's position in a girl's education and will see more in the coming chapters. In this one instance, it is likely that we see a young woman's coming to herbal knowledge *at the same time* as she comes to writing. She thus begins to own the herbal through that writing *and* that reading. The nature of the book she writes in distinguishes her signature from instances of such handwriting practice in which the young woman writes in household manuscripts, devotionals, and pleasurable print texts as recorded by Margaret Ezell, Bill Sherman, and Edith Snook, respectively.[64] As a result, Ann Parsons's signature not only gives evidence of her literacy and education but also suggests the topic of that education.. We do not know how far she went in that education or what level of literacy she reached, but her signature prompts us to reconsider other instances that we have seen.

---

64 See n. 61, above.

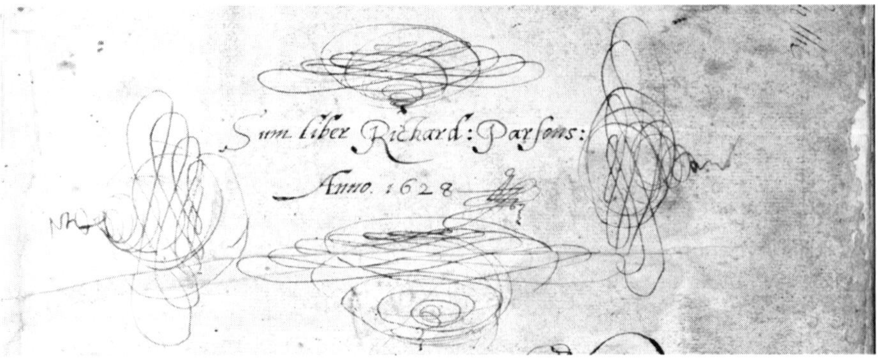

Fig. 2.8a Ownership inscription by Richard Parsons dated 1628. Rembert Dodoens, *A Nevv Herbal*, 1619, second flyleaf recto, NYPL *ZKC1410-6987. By permission of the New York Public Library.

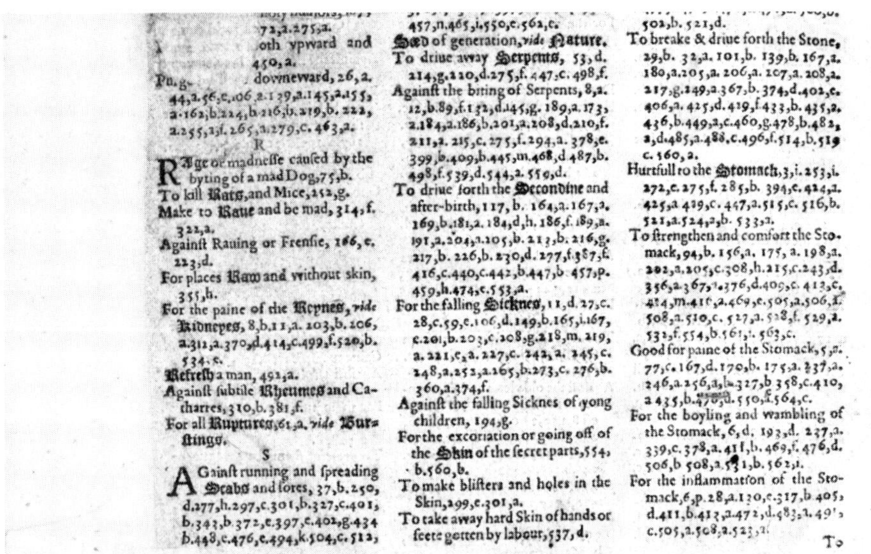
72,a.275,a.
oth vpward and 450,a.
downeward, 26,a. 44,a.56,c.106,a.139,a.145,a.155, a.162,b.224,b.216,b.219,b.222, a.255,a,f.265,a.279,c.463,a.

R

Rage or madnesse caused by the byting of a mad Dog,75,b.
To kill Rats,and Mice,252,g.
Make to Raue and be mad, 314,f. 322,a.
Against Rauing or Frensie, 166,e. 223,d.
For places Raw and without skin, 355,h.
For the paine of the Reynes, vide Kidneyes, 8,b.11,a. 203,b.206, a.312,a.370,d.414,c.499,f.520,b. 534,c.
Refresh a man, 492,a.
Against subtile Rheumes and Catharres, 310,b.381,f.
For all Ruptures,61,a. vide Burstings.

S

Against running and spreading Scabs and sores, 37,b.250, d.277,h.297,c.301,b.327,c.401, b.343,b.372,e.397,c.402,g.434 b.448,c.476,c.494,k.504,c.512,

457,n.465,i.550,e.562,c.
Seed of generation, vide Nature.
To driue away Serpents, 53,d. 214,g.220,d.275,f.447,c.498,f.
Against the biting of Serpents, 8,a. 12,b.89,f.152,d.145,g.189,a.173, a.184,a.186,b.201,a.208,d.210,f. 211,a.215,c.275,f.294,a.378,e. 399,b.409,b.445,m.468,d.487,b. 498,f.539,d.544,a.550,d.
To driue forth the Secondine and after-birth,117,b.164,a.167,a. 169,b.181,a.184,d,h.186,f.189,a. 191,a.204,a.205,b.213,b.216,g. 217,b.226,b.230,d.277,f.387,f. 416,c.440,c.442,b.447,b.457,p. 459,h.474,c.553,a.
For the falling Sicknes, 11,d.27,c. 28,c.59,e.106,d.149,b.165,i.167, e.201,b.203,c.208,g.218,m.219, a.221,e,a.227,c.242,a.245,c. 248,a.252,a.265,b.273,c.276,b. 360,a.374,f.
Against the falling Sicknes of yong children, 194,g.
For the excoriation or going off of the Skin of the secret parts,554, b.560,b.
To make blisters and holes in the Skin,299,e.301,a.
To take away hard Skin of hands or feete gotten by labour,537,d.

502,b.521,d.
To breake & driue forth the Stone, 29,b.32,a.101,b.139,b.167,a. 180,a.205,a.206,a.207,a.208,a. 217,g.249,a.367,b.374,d.402,c. 406,a.425,d.429,f.433,b.435,a. 436,b.449,a,c.460,g.478,b.482, a,d.485,a.488,c.496,f.514,b.519 c.560,a.
Hurtfull to the Stomack,3,i.253,i. 272,c.275,f.285,b.394,c.424,a. 425,a.429,c.447,a.515,c.516,b. 521,a.524,a,b.533,a.
To strengthen and comfort the Stomack,94,b.156,a.175,a.198,a. 202,a.205,c.308,h.215,c.243,d. 356,a.367,a.376,d.409,c.413,c. 414,m.416,a.469,e.505,a.506,f. 508,a.510,c.527,a.528,f.529,a. 532,f.554,b.561,i.563,c.
Good for paine of the Stomack,5,a. 77,c.167,d.170,b.175,a.237,a. 246,a.256,a,b.327,b.358,c.410, a.435,b.470,d.550,f.564,c.
For the boyling and wambling of the Stomack, 6,d.193,d.237,a. 339,c.378,a.411,b.469,f.476,d. 506,b.508,a.531,b.562,i.
For the inflammation of the Stomack,6,p.28,a.120,e.317,b.405, d.411,b.413,a.472,d.483,a.491, c.505,a.508,a.523,a.
To

Fig. 2.8b Signature of "Ann Parso[n]s," found in the "Table of the Nature, Vertues, and Dangers." From the same 1619 Dodoens, NYPL *ZKC1410-6987, sig. 3E3v. By permission of the New York Public Library.

Her Herbal, Her Authority

While much of what I have articulated here may be said of inscriptions in general, not just by women and not just in herbals, I would now like to consider what the added implications are when an inscription is by a woman and it is in an herbal. First, what we learn from these inscriptions is that the acquisition of herbal knowledge through the text is not necessarily matrilineal nor is it homosocial. Three of the four main examples above and many of the subsidiary ones include the presence of one or more men in the transfer of herbals from generation to generation and, with that transfer, the conveyance of herbal knowledge. Early modern women could inherit an herbal from a father, father-in-law, uncle, brother, or husband and could leave it to a son. Thus the introduction of the authoritative text undoes any assumed binaries of matrilineal/oral and patrilineal/textual that may exist in early feminist analyses of medical knowledge.[65] It also confirms what scholars interested in medical recipe books have discovered about the exchange of recipes between individuals of both genders.[66] This female and male collaboration reflects back on the entry from John Gerard that refers to the experiments Anne Wilbraham shared with him and anticipates our discussion of Hoby and Mildmay below.

Secondly, we may learn from these examples that the herbal is both individually and socially owned. Because of the benefits provided to the larger community, the herbal belongs to the household at large at the same time it belongs to the person who signs her name. Ann Burton's loan to "the House" is directly reflective of this, but also Ann Parsons's handwriting practice, Katherine Shirley's position in the Ferrers line, and Arthur Stacie's garden sketch all point to the household surrounding the individual. This insight is related to Lena Cowen Orlin's understanding of the closet as not necessarily a closed space, and with Orlin and Brayman Hackel, we may thus go beyond a sense of private ownership and private reading.[67] This

[65] See those examples discussed in the introduction, Jeanne Achterberg, *Woman as Healer* (Boston: Shambhala Press, 1991); Barbara Ehrenreich and Deirdre English, *Witches, Midwives, and Nurses: A History of Women Healers* (Old Westbury, New York: The Feminist Press, 1973).

[66] Sara Pennell, "Perfecting Practice? Women, Manuscript Recipes, and Knowledge in Early Modern England," *Early Modern Women's Manuscript Writing: Selected Papers from the Trinity Trent Colloquium*, ed. Victoria E. Burke and Jonathan Gibson (Aldershot, Hampshire: Ashgate Publishing, 2004), 237–58; Elaine Leong, "Note-Taking, and the Transmission of Lay Medical Knowledge" (paper presented at the meeting of the Renaissance Society of America, Cambridge, England, April 7–9, 2005); Catherine Field, "'Many hands hands': Writing the Self in Early Modern Women's Recipe Books," *Genre and Women's Life Writing in Early Modern England*, ed. Michelle M. Dowd and Julie Eckerle (Burlington, Vermont: Ashgate Publishing, 2007), 49–64.

[67] Orlin, "Gertrude's Closet"; Brayman Hackel, *Reading Material.*

social aspect of the attainment of herbal knowledge is very important in the works considered in the next two chapters.

It is clear in all of these works that texts do not appear in a woman's library in a social vacuum. Often, as is the case of Anne Purefoy and Ann Burton, books come into a woman's possession as a gift or, as in the case of Madam Burton or Sister Stacie, as a piece of inheritance. Even when a woman makes a specific purchase, as with Mary Ellys, the bought text may come with a certain set of associations. If the woman buys an authoritative herbal new and immediately from the booksellers, we can only assume, given the expense of the text, that she does so with particular purpose. In the herbals that emphasize medical experiment and value, that purpose is likely to be in medical practice, which is, in its nature, a social endeavor.

Even though our final point here may seem most obvious, it must be said: the woman who denotes her ownership of the herbal does so in order to communicate her acquisition of a certain field of knowledge. Owning the book and the knowledge it contains, and in informing others that she is its possessor, the inscriber tells others that she ultimately is the source of the expertise that they may need. Whether or not someday she will be consulted by others depends on the publicity of that knowledge, but at the very least, that knowledge is communicated within the place she lives and very likely within her circle of acquaintance. Often, and we will see this in the cases of Mildmay and Isham, other books that are owned by the woman add to the knowledge found in the herbal and testify to her concerted acquisition of medical knowledge. One hope I have for my research recorded here is that these examples may serve as a basis in the articulation of women's medical libraries.[68]

The ubiquity of these signatures and their potential for uncovering women's medical libraries gives evidence of the cultural legitimation of this knowledge for women and of the regularity with which they pursued it. We may thus add these archival findings to those uncovered by Doreen Evenden Nagy, Lucinda McCray Beier, and many others, further establishing early modern women's medical practice.[69] Again, however, my interest is in textual history, the ways in which the textual tradition frames women's participation and how women, in owning the text, both inhabit and complicate that textual construction.

So most importantly, a woman's signature in an authoritative herbal problematizes any attempts to fix medical authority within any licensing body or even within the text itself. In a sense, the signature dislocates any authority articulated through the book and shows how the circulation of knowledge places that authority within any given reader, any given practitioner. It is the context surrounding the individual woman that determines the particular nature and the extent of her appropriated authority. The more that this context is known—and

---

[68] See Laroche, "Catherine Tollemache's Library."

[69] Nagy, *Popular Medicine*; Lucinda McCray Beier, *Sufferers and Healers: The Experience of Illness in Seventeenth-Century England* (London: Routledge & Kegan Paul, 1987). See my introduction for a more complete list of historians involved in the articulation of women's roles in medical history, n. 4.

the greater awareness we have of its construction—the better we can understand the individual's relationship to medical authority, as she takes authority on herself through the text and as she acknowledges it or rejects it in others.

My analysis in the next chapter continues to explore the effect that a particular personal and family history may have on an author's representation of her acquisition of and relationship to medical authority. The elements of herbal ownership found in the signatures—male and female collaboration, one's position within a larger community, and an individual's varying pursuit of herbal knowledge alongside or against other endeavors—remain consistent threads. These elements in the sustained narratives of Margaret Hoby (1570/71–1633), Grace Mildmay (1552–1620), and Elizabeth Isham (1608/9–1654) reflect different colors and textures as they are thus examined. In each of these narratives, the herbal has an existence beyond a simple position in a trunk or on a shelf. As in Anne Clifford's triptych, the herbal gains a place within the representation of a life, and in this representation, the herbal is "owned," i.e., incorporated into the psyche and the life; the knowledge and practice it represents thus infuses the writings. We can thus go beyond fragmentary pieces of writing and beyond the material object. We can see more directly how herbal texts inform the representation of individual lives and in turn how the texts are transformed as signifiers by the context of those lives.

Chapter 3
Gentlewomen's Herbal Readings and the Absent–Present Physicians

In the previous chapter, we saw how the general signifier "herbal" moves from the more specific "Gerard's herbal" or "Parkinson's herbal" to the very specific signification "Elizabeth Bagot's herbal" or "Anne Whitehall's herbal" and how, with this last layer of designation, the text may be located not only in time/geography but within a social network as well. In this chapter, the herbal gains an even more refined location within certain life-narratives, giving it a place geographically, temporally, and socially as well as instilling it with multivalent narrative significance. The autobiographical context that provides a sense of patient and practitioner (sometimes one and the same) and remedy and disease gives narrative weight to the herbs themselves. So while Parkinson tells his female reader in the *Paradisus* that crane's bill is good for salving wounds, Lady Margaret Hoby, when confronted by a severe cut on a workman's leg, reads an herbal for just such a remedy. When Lady Grace Mildmay reads Turner's herbal and discovers that betony is good for the eyes, she combines it with other such simples to make her own unique eye medicine. When Elizabeth Isham's sister Judith suffers from melancholia and an agitated and weak heart, Elizabeth makes her a conserve from borage, which we find from the herbals is imbued with curative qualities for such ailments. Thus crane's bill, betony, and borage—all of which have other uses—have particular purpose with relation to the respective narratives. Similarly, the herbals as texts represented in these narratives come to have particular signification.

This chapter posits that, in these polysemous writings, the presence of the herbal treatises functions intertextually. As significant as the appearance of a volume of Ovid on the Shakespearean stage, the herbal texts as represented by these gentlewomen reflect upon the purposes, sources, and consequences of their writing. Two of the manuscripts to be examined in this chapter, Margaret Hoby's diary and Grace Mildmay's written legacy to her daughter and grandson, are better known and have received relatively wide commentary because they have been edited and published, thus being made generally available to a community of scholarly readers. As yet, however, the coincident presence of an herbal in the manuscripts has been read only as an extension of the regular medical practice they record. The third example, the autobiography of Elizabeth Isham, now the focus of a British online editing project,[1] further complicates the equation of herbal ownership with regular medical practice and provides an alternative understanding of early modern health care. With all three examples, I consider the writing surrounding the moments of herbal reading as the best indicator of each reading's function.

That is, despite the coincidence of herbal reading depicted in their pages, these three lives are very separate narratives, and the differences between them will contribute to subtleties in analysis. Sharon Seelig's *Autobiography and Gender in Early Modern Literature: Reading Women's Lives, 1600–1680*, with its articulation of "how individual texts are related, and how distinguished from each other," provides an elegant model for delineating generic difference within women's autobiographical texts.[2] In part these generic differences account for the diverse ways in which the herbal is represented; a central part of my analysis, moreover, works to push these differences even further and consider how variances within marital and familial status, despite similar economic backgrounds, may also contribute to our understanding. Hoby's position as a thrice-married woman without children examining her own spiritual health, Mildmay's as matron considering her own death, and Isham's as an unmarried woman providing background to her important life decisions—these differences in the purpose of the works, along with variances in age and status, inform the herbal's role in the narrative and the woman's coming to the herbal in the presentation of her life. Because of the nature of the herbal texts, this analysis of women's reading relates to but differs from those studies by Sasha Roberts and Edith Snook regarding erotic poetry and prose romance respectively, and as with their work, the insights to be gained are various and far-reaching.[3] As the many signatures suggest and these three extended manuscripts demonstrate most forcefully, there was no one way to come to herbal reading, and each individual's way was determined by her surroundings.

Key figures in the authors' milieux, especially in the consideration of the question of herbal reading, were the physicians with whom the author or her family consulted (importantly, could afford to consult) in the course of the self-narratives. How the author regarded these figures and how they informed the author's medical practice became central factors in the woman's reading practice. These men, as representatives of licensed medical authority, existed without,

---

1 *Constructing Elizabeth Isham, 1608–1654*, directed by Elizabeth Clarke and Erica Longfellow, http://www2.warwick.ac.uk/fac/arts/ren/projects/isham/ (accessed March 5, 2009).

2 Sharon Seelig, *Autobiography and Gender in Early Modern Literature: Reading Women's Lives, 1600–1680* (Cambridge: Cambridge University Press, 2006), 7.

3 Sasha Roberts, *Reading Shakespeare's Poems in Early Modern England* (Basingstoke, Hampshire: Palgrave Macmillan, 2003); Edith Snook, *Women, Reading, and the Cultural Politics of Early Modern England* (Aldershot, Hampshire: Ashgate Publishing, 2005).

alongside, or against the textual authority represented by the herbal, and as each narrative develops, the relationship between herbal reading and licensed medical authorities—whether it was substitutive, collaborative, or oppositional— becomes clearer. Again, the particularities of the life narrated and the purposes of the narrative itself are integral to understanding the author's relationship to medical authority. As Margaret Hoby's diary records the occurrence of a series of social interactions and private reflections, Mildmay's memoir transmits a legacy to subsequent generations, and Isham's remembrances attempt to make sense of a history of family illness, the physician necessarily plays a different role in each. In a way similar to the physician, the herbal text comes to signify beyond a general women's practice when we examine each instance of herbal reading with the broader narrative in mind.

"In steed of Doctor Brewer": Reading the Herbal in Margaret Hoby's Diary

Born to gentry parents Arthur and Thomasine Dakins in 1571, Margaret Hoby composed her diary between 1599 and 1605 while married to Sir Thomas Posthumous Hoby (1566–1644) and living in Hackness in Yorkshire (with occasional outings to York and London). Hoby's diary portrays the nonconformist education she received in the household of Henry Hastings, third Earl of Huntingdon, and the stoic quality of one who has survived two previous husbands, Walter Devereux (d. 1591) and Thomas Sidney (d. 1595).[4] Even though the diary's author remained childless, Hoby's days, as recorded in the diary, were packed with household duties, including attending to the health of those in and around Hackness.

Keeping in mind Seelig's warning, "the difficulty of interpretation—and the temptation of over-interpretation—is a problem with the diary . . . generally,"[5] I look to consider the relevant passages in the context of the extended record. That is, the particular nature of Hoby's diary informs the local meaning of the instances of herbal reading, while the broader context provided by the diary illuminates the general importance of the herbal's presence. Hoby's diary refers to the reading of "the arball" or "the Herball" three times,[6] all in the early-English calendar year

[4] Paul Slack, "Hoby, Margaret, Lady Hoby (*bap.* 1571, *d.* 1633)," rev., *Oxford Dictionary of National Biography*, Online Version (Oxford: Oxford University Press, 2004–06), http://www.oxforddnb.com/view/article/37555 (accessed June 26, 2007). See also the brief "case study" by Lucinda McCray Beier, *Sufferers and Healers: The Experience of Illness in Seventeenth-Century England* (London: Routledge & Kegan Paul, 1987), 218–24.

[5] Seelig, *Autobiography and Gender*, 28

[6] Mary Ellen Lamb, "Margaret Hoby's Diary: Women's Reading Practices and the Gendering of the Reformation Subject," *Pilgrimage for Love: Essays in Early Modern Literature in Honor of Josephine A. Roberts*, ed. Sigrid King (Tempe, Arizona: Center for Medieval and Renaissance Studies, 1999), 90.

1599—September, October, and February. With a close examination of the contexts surrounding the readings, we may better understand the purposes of representing this particular kind of text at this specific moment in the narration. While the diary gives ample evidence of Hoby's general reading practices, the instances of herbal reading are our focus here.

In considering Hoby's reading I must acknowledge another important analytical model for my interpretation: Mary Ellen Lamb's description of Lady Margaret's relationship with the minister Mr. Rhodes as a central artery of the diary, one that, she argues, determines the reading, writing, and other devotional practices described within and encapsulated by the diary.[7] I intend for my analysis to run in tandem with Lamb's in exploring another vital vein that I see within the text: Hoby's relationships with her physicians, at first Dr. Brewer and, after Brewer's death, Mr. Lister. In much the same way as Lamb discusses Hoby's reading of Greenham and Perkins in the context of her relationship with Mr. Rhodes, I would like to put the readings of the herbal in the context of her relationship with her physicians. In short, the herbal appears in the months after the accidental death of Dr. Brewer and before Lady Hoby has been able to establish fully her relationship with Mr. Lister. It is my argument that this is not merely coincidence but rather essential to our understanding of the location of the read text in the keeping of the diary.

Dr. Brewer died less than a month into the extant diary, so we have very little accounting of their relationship. Indeed, we hear of him only once while he is alive, in the entry from Saturday, August 25, 1599:

> In the morning I praied and then I wreet a Letter to Doctor Brewer and so to breakfast : after which I taked priuatly, with Mr Hoby, matters concerninge Conscience and our estates, w[hi]ch, beinge Concluded of betwene vs, I took my Coache and Came home to Hacknes, wher, after I was well Comed, I praise god, I went to praier and medetation : then I went about the house tell supper time : after supper I talked with Mr Rhodes in the garden, and then to publect praiers, and sonne after to bed.[8]

---

7 Lamb, "Margaret Hoby's Diary."

8 Lady Margaret Hoby, *The Private Life of an Elizabethan Lady: The Diary of Lady Margaret Hoby, 1599–1605*, ed. Joanna Moody (Stroud, Gloucestershire: Sutton Publishing, 1998), 9–10. In my research, I have consulted the original on microfilm, Lady Margaret Hoby, *The Diary of Lady Margaret Hoby*, Egerton Ms 2614, in *Medieval and Early Modern Women* (Marlborough, Wiltshire: Adam Matthew Publishing, 2000–2004), Reel 9. In citing the text, I have followed Joanna Moody's most helpful edition, except where I have, for the sake of consistency, included implied letters (made explicit in Moody) in brackets and replicated superscripts, or where I have indicated a divergent transcription in a footnote. Further page references included in the text.

We cannot tell from the entry the subject of the letter she writes to Brewer. It is an absent detail "perhaps as intriguing as the information Margaret Hoby's diary conveys."[9] From this and the surrounding entries, we may discern that Lady Hoby was in good health and did not seem to need Dr. Brewer's advice for physic; she has ventured to Linton to visit her mother, has spent much time walking in the gardens and courtyards, and has attended church, all of which she does not do when feeling too ill. Neither do we see Lady Hoby attending to patients at this point in the diary as we do later. Her letter would seem to be a simple correspondence, letting the doctor know of her planned Linton excursion from Hackness, perhaps, or following up on an earlier, unpreserved consultation with him. It is also the first in a series of exchanges with men in the day, maybe all of which are concerned with conscience, the letter and then the sincere conversations with Mr. Hoby and Mr. Rhodes thus serving as structuring events in the day's course.

Evidence of the friendliness between Lady Hoby and Dr. Brewer further materializes with the news of his death less than a week later, at which point Lady Hoby, in a rare occasion in the diary (the lack of such expression often noted in discussions of its genre),[10] expresses genuine grief and a crisis of faith. I quote the entry here in full because it is an exceptionally long one and bears close consideration:

> Friday 31
>
> After priuat praiers I I [sic] wrett notes in my testement after I had taken order in the house : then I eadt my break fast, and then wrought tell and walked tell dinner : then I praied priuatly, and, when I had dined, wrought tell :3: a clock : then I went alitle[11] about the house and reed of the diatt of the soule tell :5:, and then returned to priuat praier and medetacion, and so to readinge of the bible and walkinge tell supper : after which I hard of the sudden Death of Doctor Brewer, Procured by a medeson he minestred to him selfe to Cause him to sleep: I was much greued for it, because of the familiaritie I had with him, and good I had receiued from, but, after better aduice, I found the mercie and power of god shewed in openinge his eies touchinge me, and shuttinge them against him selfe, by Causinge him to haue great Care of minstringe vnto me, and so litle for his owne saftie : therefore I may truly conclude it is the Lord, and not the phisision, who both ordaines the medesine for our health and orderethe the ministring of it for the good of his children, closinge and vnclosinge the Iudgmentes of men at his pleasure : therefore let euerie on[e] phisision and pactente Call vpon the Lord for a blessinge: and then, after Lector, I was to[12] bed: (12–13)

9 Seelig, *Autobiography and Gender*, 21.

10 Seelig, *Autobiography and Gender*, 21; Moody, "Introduction," *Private Life*, li.

11 Differs from Moody edition, "a little."

12 Differs from Moody, "wen to."

In effect, this passage comments upon the work of the diary; the nature of self-administration and the relationships between God, physician, and patient upon which it reflects end up being formative concepts for much of the writing. Editor Joanna Moody notes that Lady Hoby was "frequently in discomfort or poor health," and it is this passage that comments directly on her relationship to that sickness.[13] In this entry, Lady Hoby establishes her familiarity with a medical authority at the same time that she discovers the fallibility, the very fragility, of that authority. She acknowledges the physician's role in her own health while also acknowledging the importance of self-administration. She demonstrates that the part of God the physician is essential to both the one who administers and the one ministered to, and in the case of self-administration for which the diary is a tool, these are one and the same.

The reported death of Dr. Brewer demonstrates a moment of self-administered medicine that goes awry; perhaps the doctor himself consulted an herbal before his death, searching under poppies or sleeping nightshade (belladonna) for the needed soporific virtue. In such an instance, the medicine thus becomes the problem, this being a moment of possible addiction and overdose. When Lady Hoby responds to the news, writing "let euerie on[e] phisision and pactente Call vpon the Lord for a blessinge," she acknowledges her vulnerability as both patient and physician. In self-administering, she occupies both roles, mirroring Dr. Brewer at the moment of his death. The diary exists at the nexus of that dual position. If she records her illness in order to assess her physical—and with it her spiritual—health, in the diary's accounts she is the patient in the description of illness and the doctor in the assessment thereof. Her role as healer becomes externalized when Lady Hoby then takes care of the wounds of others without the oversight of any male authority. The diary at once records the convergence of perceived illness, self-administering to that illness, and administering to others.

The death of Dr. Brewer also precipitates a moment in the life described in the diary during which Lady Hoby is at once patient and physician, of self and of others. Even though the diary records that she meets Mr. Lister, Dr. Brewer's eventual replacement, within a month of Dr. Brewer's death and "hope[s]" that "the Lord hath prouided [him] for me in steed of Doctor Brewer" (20), her lack of familiarity with this replacement means that the diary also reflects Brewer's absence until trust may be established. Indicative of this absence, for example, is the fact that, whereas she was in a seemingly regular correspondence with Dr. Brewer, such an exchange with Mr. Lister does not begin until after her second trip to York to consult with him more than six months later. It is in that six months that the herbal appears in Lady Hoby's diary entries. The particularities of the entries allow us to surmise the immediate reasons for consulting the herbal, and the larger context surrounding it, including the death of Dr. Brewer and the early stages of the relationship with Mr. Lister, adds another layer of significance. As long as

---

13 Moody, "Introduction," *Private Life*, xvi, which also comments upon the concept of God the physician in Hoby's diary.

Mr. Lister exists "in steed of Doctor Brewer," so too the herbal; the herbal is the means by which Lady Hoby can consult medical authority until she feels ready to consult the physician. In some ways, the herbal stands in for the physician, and importantly, in reading the herbal, so does Lady Hoby.

It is not clear where Dr. Brewer resided, but it is apparent that his absence was felt in more than the Hoby household. The diary does record that Dr. Brewer's substitute lived in York and lets us know that the distance from York to the Hoby estate was considerable: Lady Hoby took the journey always in two legs, first stopping in Linton. We can thus surmise that in a case of minor bodily injury or illness in Hackness and the surrounding communities, the physician's appearance was not expected, nor, given Lady Margaret's abilities, was it needed.[14] It is also clear, however, that Lady Hoby could not fulfill her role without some guidance. Even though it is possible that she read the herbal before and after (even during) the diary entries without recording it, the diary reports these readings in the months of the physician's absence. Thus on Monday, September 17, less than three weeks after Dr. Brewer's death and three days before Hoby meets Mr. Lister for the first time, we have the first documented consultation with the herbal:

> After priuat praier I saw a mans Legg dressed, took order for thinges in the house, and wrough tell dinner time : after dinner I went about the house, and read of the arball : then I tooke my Cocth and Came to Linton, wher, after I had talked a whill with my mother, examened my selfe and praied, I went to supper, and then praied publeckly, and so to bed: (18)

In this entry, the event of dressing the leg, which Lady Hoby describes in passive terms as if she only witnessed or oversaw it, heralds the reading of the herbal. Thus the early part of the entry would suggest that in reading she considers the various herbs helpful in healing future wounds such as crane's bill, mentioned above, or plantain. It may be, however, that it is the event immediately preceding the herbal's appearance, the meal and the subsequent housework, that brought about the consultation and Lady Hoby was in need of medicines herself, perhaps in aid of digestion, e.g., peppermint and fennel. Or a third possibility exists in anticipation of the visit with her mother and the tending to an undisclosed ailment, the trip to Linton being an interesting connection with the earlier letter to Dr.

---

14 Margaret Hoby may be one of the "case studies" that has led to the assumption that "people living outside towns . . . were largely reliant on informal, irregular and charitable provision, particularly parish clergy or benevolent gentlewomen," an assumption that Ian Mortimer attempts to refute in his historical survey of the physician's role in rural communities in Southern England; Ian Mortimer, "The Rural Marketplace in Southern England," *Medicine and the Market in England and Its Colonies, c. 1450–c. 1850*, ed. Mark S. R. Jenner and Patrick Wallis (Basingstoke: Palgrave Macmillan, 2007), 69. I contend that Mortimer's general observations do not disprove the specificities of Hoby's position as rural practitioner.

Brewer, and thus reading the herbal takes place "in steed" of writing such a letter. Regardless, I see this moment as directly related to the absence of Dr. Brewer in that, in consulting the herbal, she is either ministering to another or to herself, and the consultation shows care in whichever effort. In one way, the diary records this reading in the absence of the doctor, and the herbal stands in for his learned authority. In another way, the herbal reading occurs with Margaret Hoby acting *as the doctor*, who, in his various ministrations, would have had similar volumes to consult.

Despite the man's wounded leg, there is strong evidence that the consultation is a moment of self-administering in the fact that later that week she visited Mr. Lister for the first time. It is possible she made the trip because she felt unwell and in need of Mr. Lister's services, though her stay in York was not long and seems mostly social. The diary records only two meetings with Mr. Lister, one with "some other gentelmen" (20), along with a visit with the bishop and his wife, attendance at a christening, and conference with a "relegious gintelwoman" (21).[15] Mr. Lister is not mentioned again until the spring.

That fall and winter, the herbal appears two more times. In the next instance, Lady Hoby is home while her husband is away and her companion Mistress Brutnell reads to her:

> Munday the 15 day [October]
>
> After priuat prairs I did take my leave of Mr Hoby and, sonne after, went to church wher, a child beinge Babtised, I hard a sarmon : after, I Came home and wrett to Mr Hoby and my Mother, and sent away a messhinger to Linton : then I praied, and then to din[n]er : after, I wrett notes in my testement and walked, and, at 6: a clock, I examened my selfe and praied : then I hard Mrs Brutnell Read of the Herball tell supper time, after which I praied, and so went to bed: (29)

In the definite article and spelling, the reference here seems to denote more clearly Gerard's *The Herball or Generall Historie of Plantes*. The herbal thus appears as a specific text selected by two women for their mutual edification. Nothing in the passage suggests an immediate prompt for the text being read except the absence of men and the company of Mistress Brutnell. Whereas earlier in the day, Lady Hoby walked and wrote letters and biblical commentary, in the evening, she is read to; one imagines Lady Margaret with her eyes closed. In this entry, the herbal is the shared verbal ground between women. In the absence of Mr. Rhodes and Mr. Hoby and in this interim space between physicians, her woman and "the Herball" reconstitute the system of counsel and company to which Lady Hoby is accustomed. That is, Mistress Brutnell takes the seats of Mr. Hoby and Mr. Rhodes

---

15 Differs from Moody's "religious."

and the herbal occupies the position of Doctor Brewer, further establishing the substitutive role that the herbal takes in the diary entries.

The final appearance of the herbal occurs in the middle of a series of entries in which Margaret Hoby consistently records her position as healer–surgeon. In these entries, she increasingly owns this role, moving from the grammatical observer-position, the "saw a mans Legg dressed" in the earlier episode, to one actively engaged, "I . . . dressed a poore boies Legge[16] that Came to me" (58), to a practitioner taking care of two patients daily. In the documentation of the fourth day of attending to the wounded, February 2, she writes,

> After I had praied I dressed the sores that Cam to me : after, I dined and talked with som of my nieghbours' the afternone tell about 3 a Cloke : then I rede of the arball, went a bout the house, and returned to priuat praers : after, to supper, the[n] to publeck praier, and lastly to priuat (58)

One can tell how powerful this regular practice was for the diarist when, within a week, "the sores that Cam to me" become "my patientes" (59) in the diary. In those first days of intensive patient care, it makes sense that she would consult the herbal. One can imagine she looked for alternative salve-herbs, those available in February, from ones she has already considered, perhaps back in September. Importantly, she does not mention a physician. She is the caregiver, and the herbal is her counselor.

In part my claim that the herbal serves as counselor grows out of the bald fact that this is the last time we hear of the herbal in Lady Hoby's diary. I posit here that one reason for this textual absence was the increased presence of Mr. Lister in Lady Hoby's life. According to the diary, Lady Margaret spent a part of most every day in February attending to the patients, with follow-ups throughout March, indeed up until the very week she left for York on April 7, 1600 for her first extended treatment by Mr. Lister. During this visit in York, she consulted with Mr. Lister four times. In her last meeting with him, it seems that her thoughts returned to her patients. On April 17, she records that after reading religious materials and dining "w[i]th diuers others," she "talked with Mr. Lister touchinge sundrie thinges that Concerned more others then [her] selfe" (76). Four days later, she returned to Hackness, and three days after her return, she "dressed one that was hurt" (79), re-embracing the role she has temporarily vacated. Importantly, in the margins beside the same entry that records seeing this patient, she also documented her continued consultations with Mr. Lister, conceivably about "thinges that Concerned . . . others" (76); there she noted in a slightly larger hand, "I wret to Mr Lister" (79 n. 151). In returning to her practice, she also maintained her conferences with the physician.

In thus documenting her consultations with both physician and herbal, Hoby lets us know that, in the midst of her position as health caregiver, she is in need of

16 Differs from Moody's "boyes legge."

counsel, not simply for her own health but for the health of others. In some ways, her own sickness is the opportunity for her to establish trust with Mr. Lister, and it is in this capacity that Mr. Lister becomes the one with whom she confers. The diary records that, after this second visit, Lady Hoby sees Mr. Lister two more times, once again in York and once at Hackness. She also writes him from both Hackness and London and receives three letters from him while she is in London (October 9–March 18, 1600/1601). Importantly, during that London stay, she has dinner and two consultations with Dr. Lister, Mr. Lister's brother, who then stands in for the Yorkshire physician. Whereas Mr. Lister had once stood instead of Dr. Brewer, his place was then temporarily held by his southern brother. In this way, Lady Margaret has a physician in place virtually throughout the diary.

My point here is a simple one: in her roles as health caregiver and as patient, Lady Hoby maintained a relationship with a health counselor from the beginning almost to the very end of the diary. The two men who are the primary caregivers, Dr. Brewer and Mr. Lister, are central to her health maintenance. During two time periods, however, one or both of these men is decidedly absent. The more overt surrogate, Mr. Lister's physician brother, holds place while the Hobys visit London, but the other physician-substitute, the herbal, resides in Hackness Hall, in her own home. Thus the presence of the herbal at once marks Lady Hoby's dependence on and independence from licensed male medical authority. While she sustains a regular relationship with a series of physicians, those physicians, in their residence within cities, are consistently absent. This absence occasions Lady Hoby's own practice in tending to others and in self-administering, both of which, when a physician is in place, are supported by letters and occasional visits and, when one is not, the reading of the herbal.

The herbals themselves may acknowledge the expense of the physicians, stating that the books exist in part for the benefit of those whose "habilitie[s] [are not] so wealthy, as to entertaine a learned Phisition,"[17] and Margaret Hoby practiced in part to allay this expense for the poorer sort of her community and to alleviate the need for overextended physicians to travel great distances. Even though Ian Mortimer has established the presence of physicians in most every rural village in Southern districts, such a presence does not negate the necessity of a practice such as Lady Hoby's in terms of its immediacy and affordability.[18] What is more, her consultations with the physicians show how her practice, which was largely surgical, was meant to be complementary to rather than a substitution for, physician care. As I hope the above analysis shows, the more regular surrogate relationship is that between the herbal and the physician, and in reading the herbal, Hoby's role becomes more substitutive as well.

It is the nature of the diary that the herbal appears as a marker of difference in a series of events related in the daily accounts, which are "regular" as Seelig

---

17 Henry Lyte, "To the friendly and indifferent Reader," in his translation of Rembert Dodoens, *A Nievve Herball, or Historie of Plantes* (London, 1578), sig. *3r.

18 Mortimer, "Rural Medical Marketplace."

reminds us but "by no means identical from day to day."[19] It registers the actual absence of a trusted physician who is at once teacher and healer. What the herbal represents goes beyond the absence of the learned physician, however. It also provides a means for understanding the diary itself. Both the diary and the herbal become tools in administering to one's own spiritual and physical health and in this function reveal the reader of the texts, Lady Hoby herself, to be both healer and patient. The herbal, however, also serves to bring private reflection into public practice, which the consistent presence of Lady Hoby's patients, the eventual audience to her herbal reading, helps us to see. Again, although a woman may read the text while alone, the social uses of the herbal make that reading eventually public. Even if she reads to self-administer, she does so that she may be cured without the help of an outside authority.

The idea that medical performance may be aligned with public reading is an aspect of herbal texts that has yet to be explored. As the actor learns his lines, or the clergyman studies scripture, the medical practitioner rehearses healing in reading the text. We have seen this in the way Lady Hoby reads the herbal *after* having seen a patient, thus preparing for the next day's healing session, and can thus imagine that more concerted study would anticipate more rigorous and regular practice. The case of Grace Mildmay develops this last insight as her daily reading and practice join to become written legacy.

Approved Remedies: Reading the Herbal in Grace Mildmay's Written Remains

Lady Grace Mildmay's "rehearsals" take the form of acquiring and refining medical recipes throughout her life, a life that she recounts in one of the first autobiographies written by an Englishwoman. In that autobiography, Lady Mildmay, born to Sir Henry and Lady Anne Sharington circa 1552, tells the story of her girlhood education at the hands of her father's niece, Mistress Hamblyn, and the ways in which she spent her time during her marriage to the eldest son of Sir Walter Mildmay, Anthony, whom she married in 1567. Like Margaret Hoby, Lady Mildmay remained busy throughout her married days in her father-in-law's and then her husband's Northamptonshire estate, and in her retelling, her practice was quite regularized, dedicating a portion of each day to devotional, musical, and medical exercises. In this regularity, Grace Mildmay developed her understanding of physic in a way much more concerted than what we perceive in Hoby, and as biographer and editor Linda Pollock thus informs us, "Lady Mildmay practised medicine on a large, expensive, and systematic scale."[20] She then left the evidence

19 Seelig, *Autobiography and Gender*, 24.

20 Linda A. Pollock, "Mildmay, Lady Grace (c. 1552–1620)", *DNB*, http://www.oxforddnb.com/view/article/45817 (accessed June 26, 2007).

of this developed understanding to her daughter, Mary Mildmay Fane, and with Mary to her descendants.

Mildmay's written remains, which consist of a memoir, devotional meditations, and medical papers, are thus more self-conscious in their presentation of herbal reading and constitute one way in which Mildmay's text is "distinguished" from Hoby's.[21] Whereas Hoby's text is self-directed, reflecting a spiritual vigilance that is a kind of self-health care, Lady Mildmay writes her memoir for the benefit of others, specifically her progeny. As part of that inheritance, the memoir recounts the progress of the life that then frames and contextualizes the devotional and medical writings. In essence, the constructed representation of her life integrates the various parts of the written legacy into the whole so that her devotional meditations and medical papers each have a place within the inherited life and bear some relation to each other. The herbal's appearance in both the memoir and the medical papers provides a concise focus through which this process of integration may be examined.[22]

There are three records of Lady Grace reading an herbal in her extant writings, all of which point to methodical exercises in the practice of medicine. As the first of the accounts tells us, these exercises began when she was a child under the tutelage of Mistress Hamblyn, who had, as Lady Grace informs us, "good knowledge in phisick & surgerie."[23] Within a page of this testimony, Mildmay writes of Mistress Hamblyn's teaching methods and content:

---

[21] Seelig, *Autobiography and Gender*, 7.

[22] I am thankful for conversations with Kate Narveson, whose concerted work on Lady Mildmay's reading and writing practices with regard to biblical exegesis has done much to show "how . . . reading practice [is] related to . . . writing"; Kate Narveson, "Typography and Authority in Grace Mildmay's Manuscript Meditations," seminar paper presented at the meeting of the Shakespeare Association of America, San Diego, California, April 5–7, 2007. In her ongoing research, Narveson discusses an overinvestment on the part of critics in the medical papers because of contemporary appeal, but while it may be true that Lady Mildmay's medicine has received more attention in the work of Linda Pollock and Jennifer Wynne Hellwarth and in regular citations by medical and literary historians than has her devotional writing, I do believe that there is still room for considering how her medical practice also informs the representation of her life. Linda Pollock includes "10 per cent of her meditations and about 40 per cent of her medical papers," *With Faith and Physic: The Life of a Tudor Gentlewoman, Lady Grace Mildmay, 1552–1620* (New York: St. Martin's Press, 1993), 2; Jennifer Wynne Hellwarth focuses on the theme of medicine in "'Be unto me as a precious ointment': Lady Grace Mildmay, Sixteenth-Century Female Practitioner," *Dynamis* 19 (1999): 95–117. Many of the critics and historians discussed in my introduction cite Mildmay's papers.

[23] While indebted to Pollock's edition, *With Faith and Physic*, I have referred to the original in microfilm and provide the manuscript citations here. I have included Pollock's page numbers in my notes for those who would like to cross-reference. Grace Mildmay, "Meditations," Northamptonshire Studies Collection, Northampton Central Library, part 1., fol. 10 (Pollock 26). For the sake of clarity, I have had to leave the discussion of the

> And when she did see me idly disposed, shee would sett me to cipher with my penn, & to cast up and proove great sum[m]es & accomptes, & sometymes set me to wryte a supposed letter to this or that body concerning such & such things, & other tymes set me to reade in Dr Turners Herball, & in Bartholomew Vigoe . . .[24]

Mildmay's account confirms what Anne Clifford's commissioned triptych (discussed in the introduction) represents, the girlhood reading of herbals. Turner's text then becomes the basis for Lady Mildmay's later development of her own "good knowledge."

My analysis here diverges from readings before me in that I do not see Mistress Hamblyn as falling directly in line between Lady Anne Paget Sharington (Grace's mother) and her daughter, but rather I consider how the tutor adds an original strain in what becomes Mildmay's own life story, one that separates and develops that story from her mother's.[25] While it may be tempting to attribute the teacher's medical knowledge to her upbringing by Lady Sharington, Mildmay's writings (unlike the example of Anne Clifford's diaries discussed in the introduction) give us no indication of such knowledge belonging to her mother. Instead, Mildmay writes that the books she reads under her mother's direction are not William Turner's *New Herball* and Bartholomew Traheron's translation of Giovanni da Vigo; they are (and these "were the onely bookes she layed before me") "Musculus common places, the Imitation of Christ, and Mr Foxes Bookes of Martirs,"[26] all of which, along with the Bible, Lady Grace leaves to her daughter at the beginning of her devotional meditations. It is no coincidence that Mildmay embeds the biography of her mother within these meditations.[27] In this way, one can very easily see a maternal inheritance. "Grace Mildmay's mother," as Nancy Bradley Warren writes, "in particular played a key role in shaping her daughter's piety, a process in which Anne's experience, and those of her own mother, undoubtedly loomed large."[28] Lady Sharington instilled in her daughter, the future Lady Mildmay, a reading practice that became written devotional practice, which then became manifest in the literal books and notebooks left to Lady Fane.

---

marginal scriptural notations found throughout these manuscripts to the capable hands of Kate Narveson; see n. 22, above.

24 Mildmay, "Meditations," pt. 1, fol. 11 (Pollock 26).

25 Hellwarth sees a "matrix of female textual communities" here, "'Precious ointment,'" 116.

26 Mildmay, "Meditations," pt. 1, fol. 30 (Pollock 28).

27 Pollock's volume, *With Faith and Physic*, in part obscures this relationship between parts of the manuscript.

28 Nancy Bradley Warren, "Tudor Religious Cultures in Practice: The Piety and Politics of Grace Mildmay and Her Circle," *Literature Compass* 3.5 (September 2006): 1014.

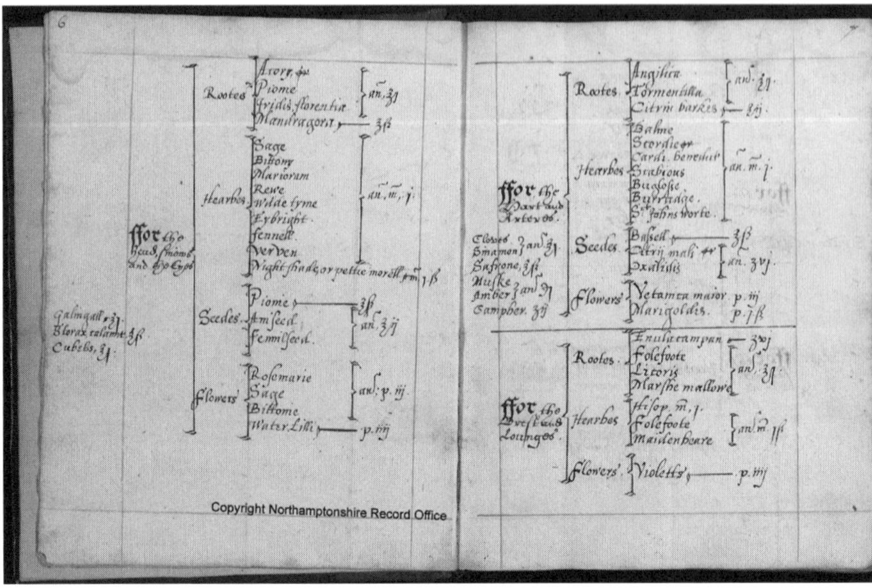

Fig. 3.1 Herbal chart from Grace Mildmay's medical papers. Northamptonshire Record Office, W(A) misc vol. 32, fols. 6–7. By permission of the Earl of Westmorland Apethorpe Settlement.

The inheritance of medical practice is not matrilineal, in that the books come from the hands of Mistress Hamblyn (not Lady Sharington), and there is no evidence that Mistress Hamblyn had received her knowledge from Lady Sharington. Instead, the only source of knowledge given is the books themselves. These texts prove to be the basis of Lady Grace's medical practice while Mistress Hamblyn provides the model for owning such knowledge and undertaking such practice. Lady Mildmay's development of these influences, however, goes beyond both the male-authored texts and the female teacher. The herbal in Mildmay's writings serves as a marker of how the author moves beyond her influences and establishes her own unique legacy.

Thus the second reference to reading the herbal shows the later development of this knowledge and practice and the further increase of Mildmay's bequest. In the memoir, Lady Grace refers to her husband's frequent absences in London and her solitude at her father-in-law's house in Northamptonshire. Lady Grace eschews the temptations of court society and frivolous company, keeping herself busy with various readings and other exercises. Among these exercises are her regular experiments and practice in medicine: "Also euery daye I spent some tyme in the Herball & bookes of phisick, & in ministring to one or other by the directions of the best phisitians of myne acquaintance, & ever god gave a blessing therevnto."[29] This entry shows a progression from the previous reference to "Dr Turners Herball"; Lady Grace maintains the childhood study presumably of Turner but no longer names Vigo (implying a focus that is not surgery),[30] and adds to the herbal other books of physic, hands-on experience, and consultations with living physicians, that last of which were more extensive than Lady Hoby's collaboration with her physicians. Lady Mildmay, it seems, knew several medical doctors, corresponding and meeting with them regularly. Her medical papers include recipes and letters from Doctors Athill, Hector, and Caudry, among others.[31] These consultations add to our understanding of the herbal's place in the attainment of such knowledge; the herbal becomes one version of medical authority from which a woman may gather her own. The autobiography demonstrates how Lady Mildmay developed her education and thus enhanced her daughter's inheritance; while she added her meditations to the devotional inheritance from her mother, she contributed her own experience and communication with the "best physicians" to the work of Turner, in effect going beyond the male-authored text while creating her own manuscripts.

Outside the autobiographical accounts, Mildmay did not mention an herbal, nor did she leave an herbal, Turner's or any other, to Mary Fane in the list of her inherited texts. What Fane did inherit, however, are the "divers books" and "more than 2,000 loose papers"[32] holding the results of Grace Mildmay's lifelong medical experience, and it is these papers that provide the third instance of Mildmay's reading of the herbal. That is, these papers contain a chart of herbs and their medicinal uses (Figure 3.1). At first glance, this chart appears to be a distillation of the larger text and could be a visually realized "epitome" comparable to what we have seen in the example of the Bulckley remedy book discussed in the introduction.[33] Upon closer examination, however, we realize that it reflects an active reading of the herbal beyond the expedient elisions and more straightforward copying the Bulckley Compiler A executes. Mildmay revises and updates her source, and one imagines that she does so through the "other books of physic," her discussions with physicians, and her experience with patients related in the autobiographical account of her early adulthood. In these writings, she does

---

29 Mildmay, "Meditations," pt. 1, fol. 46 (Pollock 35).

30 Indeed, Pollock notes that "surgery . . . is rarely dealt with in her papers," *With Faith and Physic*, 98.

31 Hellwarth writes of "actual encounters and consultations with physicians, or . . . 'consultations' with the texts by renown[ed] physicians" but does not develop this thread, "'Precious ointment,'" 109.

32 Mary Fane's "Description of Lady Mildmay's papers," transcribed by Pollock in *With Faith and Physic*, 110.

33 Compare Pollock's naming these pages "a list of herbs and flowers" then rendering them as such, *With Faith and Physic*, 103, 127–28.

not merely study or consult the text; she engages it, moving away from mere "simples" and toward complex medicinal recipes.

My analysis is based on a cross-referencing with William Turner's complete herbal, as Turner is the only herbalist identified in the account—the "the" of the second reference to "the Herball" denoting the previously named "Dr Turners Herball"—and it is this authoritative text from 1568 that would have been available in the early years of her marriage.[34] The many correspondences between the herbal virtues described by Turner and those found in the herbal chart imply that Turner's text contributes to the chart's construction; however, the very format on the page, along with the variations from Turner, shows that the author has gone beyond mere copying. Mildmay's page looks like a modern-day flowchart, with the categories "ffor the Head, Sinews, and the Eyes," "ffor the Brest and Lounges," "ffor the matrix," etc., written on the far left of the page.[35] For each of these titles, the next column bears the subcategories "Rootes," "Hearbes," "Seedes," "Flowers" (sometimes omitted), and (more rarely) "Barck" and "Spices," and each subcategory then leads to a list of one to ten plants. From these lists each plant or group of plants has its own notation, with alchemical symbols denoting units of measure such as ounces and manipules.[36] Unlike "The Booke of Hearbes & Receipts," which replicates the virtues for select individual plants (conceivably the herbs the compiler had in her fields and gardens) as they appear in Gerard's *Herball*, Mildmay catalogs the plants under the organ they can help heal. Diverging from the conventional herbal entry, this organization in and of itself shows a direct engagement with the text, especially if Mildmay continues to consult Turner throughout her life. Unlike Dodoens, Gerard, and Parkinson, Turner's herbal does not contain an index of medicinal benefits;[37] she would have had to read each entry or had relevant entries pointed out to her in order to discover that garden mint was "good for ye stomack"[38] or that betony helps with "clerenes of

---

34 I am aware here that the Turner's complete herbal of 1568 would have been late for Mildmay's childhood education, but the account of her childhood gives "The Herball" a referent. It is likely that someone of Mildmay's station and acumen could acquire subsequent volumes as they were published. While in the Hoby example, "The Herball" seems to refer directly to Gerard, the reference here seems too early a date for the newly married Mildmay to be using Gerard's text or even the 1578 Dodoens, *A Nievve Herball.*

35 The charts in question are in Mildmay's "Medical Papers," Northamptonshire Record Office available through the Earl of Westmorland Apethorpe Settlement, W(A) misc vol. 33, fols. 6, 7, and 10, respectively.

36 See Fred Getting's list of "Alchemical Weights and Measures" in Appendix 4 of his *Dictionary of Occult and Alchemical Sigils* (London: Routledge, 1981), 320.

37 As a sidenote, even if Mildmay's adulthood brought her a copy of Dodoens or Gerard, the organization still demonstrates a noteworthy level of engagement because the indexes in these later texts give only the page, not the name, of the herb.

38 William Turner, *The first and seconde partes of the herbal of William Turner Doctor in Phisick/lately ouersene/corrected and enlarged with the thirde parte/lately gathered* (Cologne, 1568), fol. 2.54r. Subsequent citations included in the text.

the eyes" (1.82). Beyond this system of organization, the individual entries show the process of revision as arrived at through cross-referencing, experimentation, or outside consultation. For example, Turner's entry for fennel records that "it is also good both for diseases of the liuer and the longues" (fols. 2.4v–2.5r). Mildmay lists fennel under the roots (Turner distinguishing little between the parts of the plants) good "for the liver" but not under herbs helpful for the lungs; this omission would seem to indicate that she had not thus found fennel useful for the lungs. What is most striking about these pages, moreover, is the way in which they move toward something beyond the individual parts. Mildmay's medicinal recipes—for example, the recipe for making "A most precious and excellent Balme" that comes directly after these charts[39]—also list the ingredients by plant parts and other medical categories such as roots, herbs, seeds, flowers, spices, gums, purgatives, and cordials. Furthermore, in the left-hand margins of the earlier pages, we can see Mildmay adding ingredients such as "cloves" and "sinamon," which often belong to a category such as "spices" that the original recipe does not include. These subsets of ingredients show how Mildmay develops her recipes in stages, adding ingredients systematically to her cure. Mildmay's flowcharts, therefore, represent complex medicinal formulae.

In this one portion of her papers, we have a metonymic representation of all two thousand plus leaves recording Mildmay's medical experiments. The herbal charts, as well as the papers in general, add years of experience and expert input to her textual study. In this way, the herbal as represented in her memoir prefigures the papers themselves; that is, her writings come to replace the male-authored texts from which she herself has learned. References to the herbal in the memoir, therefore, work metatextually within the autobiography of Lady Mildmay in the way they prefigure the writings her daughter will one day inherit. Mildmay's writings record how she develops the knowledge she garners from her teachers, either from her mother and Mistress Hamblyn or from the books they prescribe. These writings let us know that, eventually, what Mary Fane is to inherit is her mother's education, plus interest.

Thus focusing on the herbal allows us to see the metatextual potentials within Mildmay's works as one text in a series of texts becomes the foundation upon which the current manuscript evolves. Most directly, a focus on the herbal as metatext highlights for us the medicinal metaphor from the following passage, which speaks directly to the purposes of the memoir and, consequently, to her devotions:

> **This book of my Meditation** is the consolation of my soule, the joye of my hart & the stabilitie of my mynde.
>
> As they are approued by the word of God, & as I do approoue them in myne owne conscience by the same word. -----

[39] Mildmay, "Medical Papers," fol. 11.

> And I haue not sett them downe for ostentation or vanitie, as God himselfe is witnesse but with the zeale of my hart -----
>
> Knowing that there is nothing hath happened vnto me in the course of my lyfe, either in prosperity or aduersitie in any kynde whatsoeuer, but the lyke maye fall out to some other, wherein my comforts & remedies may be approued vnto them as they have been vnto me.[40]

In light of this passage, the herbal prefigures not only the "divers volumes" of medical papers but also the writings as a whole; in the context of the herbal, the written legacy becomes a kind of healing practice. The "approued" "comforts and remedies" are the practices of medicine, devotion, music, and needlework themselves, the former two being evidenced in the textual inheritance. Mildmay adds to these "remedies" lengthy accounts of the forbearance she shows against the strain of her husband's absence and the resolution of the awful filial tension transpiring after her father's death.[41] Both Warren and Hellwarth recognize the "considerable linguistic overlap between Grace's spiritual and medical texts,"[42] and this particular moment of "overlap" highlights an intertextuality that blurs generic distinction. In providing "comforts and remedies," the meditations taken from the Bible and Foxe become analogous to her medical papers, volumes that are, in turn, derived from her consultations beginning with Turner's herbal and developed through other medical texts as well as learned physicians. As the herbal provides the basis for her entire medical practice, it also provides a conceptual foundation for her writing practice as well.

Again, the juxtaposition of Lady Grace Mildmay's textual remains and Lady Margaret Hoby's diary highlights Seelig's distinguishing contexts of autobiographical writing. In Hoby's diary, the herbal illuminates the consistent but variable absent-presence of the physician that the diary in some way negotiates, while the layering of life-experience, physician consultation, and regular experiment onto the herbal in Mildmay's written remains reflects the originality and accumulation that is her life. This generic difference is accompanied by another difference, however: that of the difference between an almost-thirty childless wife in her third marriage and an older grandmother at the close of her days. Mildmay writes and preserves her texts as inheritance, and it is in this inheritance that the herbal becomes one text among the larger collection. Lady Hoby's diary, written in the now, presents the herbal as one in a series of texts related to a series of individuals that occupy her days and mind. In our third example, Elizabeth Isham's autobiography, the herbal

[40] Mildmay, "Meditations," pt. 1, fols. 30–31 (Pollock 25).

[41] Lena Cowen Orlin addresses the tensions surrounding Grace Mildmay's inheritance from her father in her essay "Chronicles of Private Life," *The Cambridge Companion to English Literature, 1500–1600*, ed. Arthur Kinney (Cambridge: Cambridge University Press, 2000), 250–52.

[42] Warren, "Tudor Religious Cultures," 1031; Hellwarth, "'Precious ointment.'"

is neither a prefigurement nor a replacement but rather represents the culmination of various influences at a moment of crisis and decision.

"Those hearbs and flowres which I had wrought": Reading the Herbal in Elizabeth Isham's *Booke of Rememberance*

Like Lady Hoby and Lady Mildmay, Elizabeth Isham was of the landed gentry to "was a gentlewoman from an influential family and left a written account of her life. Her father was Sir John Isham (1582–1651), first baronet, and her mother was Judith Lewyn Isham (d. 1625). Her brother Justinian would become second baronet and father of four daughters who survived infancy; her sister Judith died in her mid-twenties. Throughout most of her time on earth, Elizabeth lived in the family estate of Lamport Hall in Northamptonshire, but on occasion she visited her relatives, the Dentons and the Pagets, in London. In pointed contrast to Hoby and Mildmay, however, Elizabeth Isham never married, and this fact proves to be one of the most important aspects of her life as she described it.[43] Also, Isham's autobiographical account does not describe an extensive medical practice. It does, however, show another way in which a woman may have come to have read an herbal: not in her girlhood education and developing sense of scientific inquiry or in her established position as country practitioner, but rather in an independent and multiply motivated pursuit of one kind of knowledge over another.

Dated 1638/39 by the *Constructing Elizabeth Isham* collective, the quarto-sized manuscript constituting *My Booke of Rememberance* [*sic*] is made up of thirty-eight leaves written in a small, accomplished italic hand. Defining features of the document are the extensive marginalia throughout, most of which seem to have been written during sessions later than the writing of the main body of the text.[44] The manuscript meditates upon Isham's life crises and moments of fateful

---

43 For an extended discussion of Isham's various suitors and the nature of her decision, see Isaac Stephens, "The Courtship and Singlehood of Elizabeth Isham, 1630–1634," *The Historical Journal* 51.1 (2008): 1–25.

44 For the sake of continuity and space, in the quotations to follow I have either inserted bracketed ellipses or the bracketed marginal note in the appropriate place. In determining the position of these brackets, I have most often followed the decisions of Alice Eardley, the transcriber for the autobiography in the *Constructing Elizabeth Isham* project. While most indebted to Eardley's transcription, for consistency with the rest of this study, I have not denoted linebreaks, but I have tried, through superscripts and ampersands, to emulate the compact quality of Isham's writing; Alice Eardley's transcription, in "Elizabeth Isham's Lives," makes most of the Princeton manuscript available online, http://www2.warwick.ac.uk/fac/arts/ren/projects/isham/ (accessed March 4, 2009). My thanks to the directors, Elizabeth Clarke and Erica Longfellow, for inviting me to participate in this project at its initial stages. Some of the general observations expanded on in this chapter are outlined in the collaborative essay, Michelle DiMeo and Rebecca Laroche, "Elizabeth Isham and Medicine," found linked to that site, http://www2.warwick.ac.uk/fac/arts/ren/projects/

decisions, always with deference to an immediate divine audience and an eye to an ultimate familial readership in her brother and his children. The moment from the autobiography in which she records setting the course to read the herbal occurs late in the narrative, after the death of her grandmother and mother, after an extended stay in London, after she has decided to remain unwed, and after her sister Judith's always unstable health has worsened. Isham writes of this time in her mid-twenties,

> Now I had a mind to learn latin, wch because I could . . . not so well compasse (by reason of [. . .] other accations) Therefore I rather tooke holde of S pauls words \I cor. 8./1. Knowledge puffeth [. . .] up. but love edifieth. I therefore purposed to read of y^{e} vertue of those hearbs & flowres which I had wrought, wch as they are different in there shapes & coullers so are there vertues: which made me often call to mind y^{e} 24 verse of y^{e} 104 psalme. O Lord how manifold are thy workes: in wisdome hast thou made them all: I found this way might be very beneficiall both to my Sister & others. & y^{t} I might make ye best use of those things w^{ch} [. . .] our garden afforded. wch abounded in those things wch was cordiall for her | [45]

After the vertical mark, the passage continues "as rosmary, roses" and follows a diagonal line into the right hand margin to "& borrage wch I made conserues of &c" (fol. 28r). A related document in the Northamptonshire archives, a kind of memory chart that reconstructs events in Isham's life by year, reveals that Isham did read "of the vertue of hearbs" in 1633 and before this moment, she had turned to "a booke which my Sister borrowed of Gardening."[46] We also know that her decision to pursue this knowledge meant that she eventually turned to an actual herbal because of another piece of evidence, a book inventory found on the back of a 1648 letter from an aunt, which includes the unnumbered entry, "An Herball," above the numbered entry 42, "A book of gardening."[47] Which specific herbal this

isham/medicine/ (accessed February 12, 2009). See also, Isaac Stephens's transcription, http://history.ucr.edu/people/grad_students/stephens/TheAutobiography.pdf (accessed February 12, 2009).

[45] Elizabeth Isham, "Autobiography, ca. 1640s," Robert H. Taylor Collection, Princeton University Library, RTC01 no. 62, fol. 28r. Subsequent citations included in the text. Isham, "Book Inventory," Northamptonshire Records Office, IC 4829; my thanks to Jill Millman for sharing her transcription before I was able to see the digital image.

[46] "Northamptonshire Diary," Northamptonshire Records Office, IL 3365; for this reference I am dependent on Jill Millman's transcription (e-mail to the author, August 13, 2007) and the *Constructing Elizabeth Isham* collective.

[47] For another book inventory that lists a copy of Gerard's herbal amongst its holdings, see for comparison *The Southwell–Sibthorpe Commonplace Book: Folger MS. V.b. 198*, ed. Jean Klene (Temp, Arizona: Medieval & Renaissance Texts & Studies, 1997), 99–101. As it lists its books in order of size, the Southwell–Sibthorpe manuscript lists the herbal as one of its first items.

is remains a point of discussion, but one thing is certain: she articulates here her choice to pursue herbal knowledge over the learning of Latin.

Within the autobiography, she has displayed an inclination toward the latter in her account of her London stay with the Pagets, during which her Aunt Denton wanted her to learn French in her "recreation" as many women in London society; however, Isham "had . . . more mind to latten thinking it more profitable," and her cousin Thomas Paget had a compassionate inclination to teach her (fol. 20v). Her lessons did not progress "further then ye declensions of pronounes" because of many other pursuits, but this account anticipates the later decision to choose herbalism over Latin, letting us know some history behind the decision (fol. 20v). Her position as a woman not allowed to enter the university and dependent on the time of male associates explains why Elizabeth could "not so well compasse" Latin in the later moment when such male beneficence is less available, and in this light, her invocation of scripture may seem to be a rationalization denying her real desire.

On the surface, Elizabeth Isham's choice to forgo Latin so as not to appear too "puffed up" seems motivated by gender constructs and expectations in which women did not learn Latin but could study medicine. Such gender restrictions have been well deconstructed by the work of Jane Stevenson, which shows the extensive knowledge of Latin held by gentlewomen in the period,[48] and a closer examination of the episode itself with relation to the larger autobiography reveals how the narrative of gender educational inequities may oversimplify the complexities of her decision. The passage identifies several impetuses behind the resolution, not the least of which is her sister's health. This passage ultimately cites this anxiety-producing factor after it alludes to Isham's position in the country estate (away from the educated and educating society of London), the continuities with her most pleasurable pastime in needlework, and the grounding in biblical precedent. The larger autobiography also delineates the filaments of family history—a mother long ill and little able to care for her daughters, an aunt and great-grandmother with notable skills in medicine, and a growing household distrust of physicians—that led to the certainty of Elizabeth Isham's choice.

The history of illness in the Isham household may very well prove to be the largest determining factor in Elizabeth's decision to pursue herbalism. Aside from a series of painful bone breaks experienced by her younger sister and the final illness of a grandmother, the early part of the autobiography is dominated by her mother's chronic poor health throughout the author's girlhood and the mother's eventual death apparently from pneumonia or consumption when Elizabeth was only sixteen. The long-term illness itself is difficult for us to diagnose, but the overriding symptoms are a weakness of limbs, extreme menstrual bleeding, an often consuming depression, a susceptibility to communicable diseases, and for a time, a palsy in the tongue. At various moments in the narrative, the mother's

---

[48] Jane Stevenson, *Women Latin Poets: Language, Gender, and Authority, from Antiquity to the Eighteenth Century* (Oxford: Oxford University Press, 2005).

sickness reaches a crisis point, and at these times, a seeming army of physicians and surgeons descends on the Isham household, the most memorable of such moments occurring when the eldest daughter is still a young girl of nine or ten:

> now the time . . . came in which my mother was to haue those meanes for her hea[l]th ministred unto her, which was in a maner [. . .] a whole course of phisyck as first 3 vomits within few dayes one of another. then \a/ potion \(twise)/ after a decoction & pilles. w^{t} letting of bleed in y^{e} arme, and gargarismes also y^{e} phisycions agreed that her hare should be cut, hauing quilted capps for her w^{t} herbs of hot nature, [which were in her meats, and drinkes as Rosemary, sage,marg\e/rome, bitonie, sassafrus in her drinke] w^{t} perfumes to fume them over, all these she suffered w^{t} cuting of her hare. which was both fare \coloured/ and long, yet after the growth of it & leting of blood in the tongue w^{t} cordialls, & exorcise, wch she was much perswaded unto, [& sweting] she after mended by degrees praised be God: (fol. 14r)

In throwing every possible treatment at the patient (many of which were violent and invasive), this medical surge must have made an impact on the observant young girl. Indeed, the poignant cutting of the mother's hair intercedes between the healing and the most aggressive treatments, only the "leting of blood in the tongue" coming after that dramatic and most fully realized treatment of the "quilted capps." Even though this medical heavy-handedness would appear to have had the desired effect in the mother's mending "by degrees," Isham's syntax here attributes the most worth to the cordials and exercise at the end of the list.

My reading of this passage's sentence structure in part grows out of the persistent inefficacy of the physicians who take care of Lady Isham and the resulting expressions of distrust in Elizabeth's accounts of their treatments. The passage of the vomiting and haircutting occurrence anticipates the record of the mother's decision to do without the "taking of phisicke" for two or three years (fol. 17v) and of her "moane" to her sister-in-law in the last weeks of her life that "she had suffered many things of physitions" (fol. 19r). At this later moment in Isham's account, both mother and daughter (in quoting her mother) allude to the biblical passage in Mark (5.26) that describes a woman whose problem with nonstop menstrual bleeding had left her not only weak and despairing but also financially bereft.[49] Also, in this final stage of her mother's illness, Elizabeth observes that when he was sent for, "her olde Physitian Mr Langam" did not attend her mother, saying "he had no hope of doeing her good" (fol.19r). Her so-minuscule-as-to-be-almost-hidden marginalia reveal much here; the marginal note's position by this passage, "hoping to live," applies that comment more readily to Mr. Langham, who fears contagion, not to the mother, who is at peace with her own demise at

[49] My thanks to Harold Vanderpool at the Institute for the Medical Humanities at the University of Texas Medical Branch for bringing the specificity of this allusion to my attention.

this point, nor to the father, who sends for the doctor. This reading is supported by Mr. Langham's decision at the time not to "medle" with the sister's illness either (fol. 19r). It seems that, up until her death, Lady Isham had little to be thankful for in her physicians.

In the narrative, this faulty diagnosis and mistrust continues beyond the mother's death into the sister's treatment. One crisis moment records how "the cause of her illnesse was said to be ye mother [the womb] but those things wch was proper for the desease availed not neither did other sircumstances a gree w^{t} ye phisitians rule for it" (fol. 22r). Again, Isham's syntax is particularly revealing here, as the passive voice at first puts "the cause of her illnesse" in an authoritative voice, as if the cause was given from on high, but as the sentence progresses, "ye phisitians rule" proves to be false. So the accounts of the mother's and sister's flawed—often invasive—treatments by licensed medical authorities communicate mistrust and ground it in biblical precedent. This suspicion markedly contrasts with the spirit of collaboration seen in the Hoby and Mildmay writings (although perhaps such suspicion is hinted at in the account of Dr. Brewer's death). With this expressed distrust in mind, we may read Elizabeth Isham's turn to herbal knowledge as a means of offsetting the faults of physician care.

Buttressing this movement away from licensed medical authority is the often benevolent and beneficial care of alternative practitioners given toward the mother's and sister's health. As Lucinda McCray Beier notes, Lady Hoby also "consulted other healers," but they seemed in supplement to, not as replacement for, the physician.[50] At one point in Isham's narrative, Lord and Lady Isham decide to confer with "Mr. Naper," "comanly called Sandy," who was known for his "good skill in physick," but who Lady Isham "feared" "used inderict meanes" (fol. 18v). Erica Longfellow has posited that this is none other than Richard Napier, the famous astrologer and physician, who was "abused by some as a conjuror or witch."[51] The summoning of the family minister to go to Mr. Napier to retrieve the cordials he prescribes implies that Sandy's practice did have the taint of witchcraft and the Ishams feared irreligious influence. Despite the irregular source for the medicines, his cordials brought about a recovery that had Judith Isham living throughout another year. Similar to this episode is a later one involving Elizabeth's sister, who asked for the help of a female servant of a neighbor Mr. King, "of whom she had some helpe afore & . . . gessed nearer her illness, then ye phisitian" (fol. 29v). In a manner following the way the Ishams sent their minister to Napier to offset supernatural affiliations, Isham's narrative reveals anxiety about at least the perception concerning non-physician care when she concludes this account with the caveat, "though not by y^{t} meanes wch is contrary to thy word for both my

---

50 Lucinda McCray Beier, *Sufferers and Healers*, 222.

51 Erica Longfellow speaking at the workshop *Constructing Elizabeth Isham*, Princeton University, September 7–8, 2007. Quotation taken from Jonathan Andrews, "Napier, Richard (1559–1634)," *DNB*, http://www.oxforddnb.com/view/article/19763 (accessed January 7, 2008).

selfe & \my/ sister hated all fauls waies," adding in the margins "& divers times wee perswaded our people y^{t} they should not goe to wiches or wisards" (fol. 29v). These two episodes of alternative medical practice demonstrate how disspelling the shadow of witchcraft from efficacious but socially suspect medical care may be another motivation for the devout Elizabeth Isham to take on her own practice.

As seen in the Napier episode, a common ingredient of beneficial care seen in the autobiography is the cordial, or "a medicine, food, or beverage which invigorates the heart and stimulates the circulation."[52] The narrative relates that, along with the improvement seen in the mother on various occasions as a result of cordials, the one physician who seems to have helped the younger Judith when she was taken ill soon after and because of her mother's death "gave her a cordiall & other things" (fol. 21v), and when it was believed that she "should haue died," she seemed "to haue the most comfort (of y^{t} she tooke) of cordialls complaining much of her heart saying it was as if it were sooden w^{t} in her" (fol. 22r). Before this episode, Elizabeth Isham records her belief that "my mothers taking of many cordials so fortified her nature wch made her have ye greater combat w^{t} death for she would often say if she had bin a poore woman she had died long afore this" (fol. 19v). Alongside the general concerns about her sister's health expressed as part of the decision to turn to herbalism is the more specific interest in a particular kind of medicine, "those things which [were] cordial for her" (fol. 28r). In that later entry, Elizabeth Isham emphasizes "cordial" not only as a liqueur (with admitted alcoholic potentials) but also as an adjective, that is, a quality, not simply a form, of medicine. In this quality, the medicines that seemed to have helped both mother and daughter are described as gentler than the invasive or purgative and often violent treatments proposed by many of the physicians depicted in the memoir. Indeed, liquid cordials are afforded a kind of magical efficacy in the narrative, and more important than the gentle liqueurs are the non-purgative and calming aspects of the herbs at the foundation of the medicines.

In concert with witnessing the benefits of cordials, Elizabeth Isham's desire to make such medicines may also grow out of her familial inheritance from her Aunts Isham and her paternal great-grandmother. An "Aunt Isham," whether the wife to her Uncle Henry or her Uncle Richard or both women (as "they both liued in ye toune" close to Lamport Hall [marginalia fol. 11r]), plays a role throughout the narrative. Elizabeth describes Henry's wife as "a fitt woman to minister helpe" to Judith Isham "both for her mind & body" and the other Aunt Isham as a "vertuous woman" (fol. 11r). As the latter is introduced to us as being ill herself and only the former receives the label of healer, it is likely Henry's wife that attended the mother Judith and conferred with the girls at moments of health crisis. Regardless, it is one Aunt Isham who sits with her sister-in-law in her final illness.

It is also an Aunt Isham that orients Elizabeth to her medicinal inheritance during arguably one of the most influential moments in Elizabeth's decision to

---

52 "cordial, n^{1}," *The Oxford English Dictionary*, 2nd ed. 1989, *OED Online*, Oxford University Press, http://dictionary.oed.com/cgi/entry/50050112 (accessed March 2, 2009).

pursue herbal knowledge. The account is of a moment when she is twenty-four and Elizabeth experiences "a paine in [her] right thigh" that is "like ye paine or griping of ye wind collicke" (fol. 26v). As it is told, the young woman finds a cure, interestingly enough, in her own closet, where she discovers a vial of forty-year-old "oiles of swallowes" (fols. 26v–27r), possibly swallowwort oil, that was "of [her] Great Granmother Ishams making, who was . . . very skilful in Surgery & did many charitable deeds y^{t} way" (fol. 27r).[53] The memoir records how her Aunt Isham, "who knew what belonged to such things," encouraged Elizabeth to use it as it may have retained some "vertue." This oil, when combined with exercise, caused the pain "to be somthing eased" (fol. 27r). In understanding this inheritance, it may help us to note that Isham's late Tudor great-grandmother would have been within one generation of Lady Grace Mildmay; thus preserved, the oil represents a thing of the past, yet one that still has some use and importance. Three generations removed, Elizabeth Isham's practice, surrounded by physicians, would doubtlessly have a different cultural currency.

While the answer would be nearly impossible to determine completely, this instance begs us to ask how it may reflect a change in women's medical practice because of the presence of the text. One wonders if Isham's great-grandmother, or even her aunt for that matter, needed to "read of ye virtue[s] of those hearbs" to know the healing powers of plants (fol. 28r). Rebecca Tannenbaum has speculated on the growing influence of textual medicine in her study of colonial women's practice,[54] and we may similarly speculate that the presence of the text made medicinal knowledge less immediate and something that has to be recaptured through those very texts and through concerted questioning of the previous generation. Isham did not get herbal knowledge from her mother, who is noted on the first page of the narrative to decidedly shun such pursuits early in her life (marginalia fol. 2v), but the frequent visits of her aunt and books borrowed from some undisclosed source point to alternative means by which such knowledge may be obtained.

---

[53] There is a recipe for "Oyl of swallowes" in Gervase Markham, *The English Husvvife*, first published in 1615, which contains many different herbs as well as the main ingredient, here up for debate. Unlike mid-seventeenth-century print versions of the recipe, when viewed alongside plants, Markham's recipe, which includes "twenty quick Swallows" (45), leaves some ambiguity as to whether or not it includes actual live animals. The herb swallowwort contains seed pods shaped like the birds' wings, perhaps referenced in the recipe as "swallows," leaving open the possibility of a complete vegetable concoction described by Markham. Because of the focus of the Isham narrative on herbal cordials, the age of the oil, and the virtue of swallowwort to help with cramps, I am willing to preserve the idea that there was no animal abuse involved in the making of this product. I imagine the debate will continue. I have consulted the 1668 edition, Markham, *The English House-wife*, 44–45, reproduced in *Defining Gender, 1450–1910*, (Marlborough, Wiltshire: Adam Matthew Publications Ltd., 2005), http://www.gender.amdigital.co.uk/contents/image-viewing.aspx?imageid=5241 (accessed March 10, 2009).

[54] Rebecca Tannenbaum, *The Healer's Calling: Women and Medicine in Early New England* (Ithaca, New York: Cornell University Press, 2002), 141–43.

This combination of influences—the mother's and sister's prolonged illnesses, the resulting distrust of physicians, and the proved efficacy of herbal cordials and alternative care validated by the positive presence of female healers in the familial line—certainly contributed to Elizabeth Isham's resolution to abjure Latin for the study of herbs. These reasons are all quite practical, in that they give material purpose to her study. Her autobiography also provides two less pragmatic though no less immediate reasons for her decision: herbalism's relationship to the pleasures of needlework and gardening and the young woman's immersion in scripture.

Elizabeth Isham's phrasing about the moment of her decision, "to read of ye vertue of those hearbs & flowres which I had wrought," perfectly captures the symbiotic relationship between the two endeavors in her mind (fol. 28r). In line with Jennifer Munroe's analysis of the continuities between gardening and needlecraft, I propose here that the inseparability of needlework and herbalism in Isham's mind is not simply aesthetic but also textual.[55] Namely, in the Northamptonshire diary and then in her book inventory, Elizabeth Isham lists "A book of gardening." As we have seen in previous chapters, Parkinson's *Paradisi in Sole Paradisus Terrestris* facilitates an exchange between the "delights" found through plants, such as needlework and gardening, and the "use" of them in medicine, and it is very possible that the gardening book in question is the *Paradisus*, which she would have used not only for gardening instructions—one marginal note refers to her "delight" in the "seting of herbs" (fol. 19r)—but also in her needlework for which the illustrations could provide patterns. Such use of botanical book illustrations has been demonstrated by Munroe and Linda Levy Peck and further substantiated in my own findings at the Library of Congress, where eighteenth-century embroidery patterns are pressed between the pages of one copy of Parkinson's *Theatrum Botanicum*;[56] furthermore, Parkinson himself recognizes needlework patterns as one of the uses of his book, pointedly under borage, from which Isham reports making conserves for her sister.

55 Jennifer Munroe, "'In this Strang Labourinth, How Shall I Turne?': Needlework, Gardens, and Writing in Mary Wroth's Pamphilia to Amphilanthus," in *Gender and the Garden in Early Modern English Literature* (Burlington, Vermont: Ashgate Publishing, 2008), 97–120.

56 Munroe, "'In this Strang Labourinth'"; Linda Levy Peck, *Consuming Splendor: Society and Culture in Seventeenth-Century England* (Cambridge: Cambridge University Press, 2005). John Parkinson, *Theatrum Botanicum* (London, 1640), Library of Congress, QK41 .P2 Bitting Coll., copy 2; this copy includes the elegy to Mistress F. discussed in Chapter 2. See also Susan Frye, "Sewing Connections: Elizabeth Tudor, Mary Stuart, Elizabeth Talbot, and Seventeenth-Century Anonymous Needleworkers," in *Maids and Mistresses, Cousins and Queens: Women Alliances in Early Modern England*, ed. Susan Frye and Karen Robertson (New York: Oxford University Press, 1999), 165–182. Deborah Harkness offers this as a reason for gentlewomen to have bought Gerard's herbal, *The Jewel House: Elizabethan London and the Scientific Revolution* (New Haven, Connecticut: Yale University Press, 2007), 15.

Despite the medicinal value that would otherwise place bugloss and borage in the volume's "Kitchen Garden," Parkinson has placed them in his "Garden of Pleasant Flowers" and justifies his decision with the following:

> Although Borage and Buglosse might as fitly haue been placed, I confesse, in the Kitchen Garden, in regard they are wholly in a manner spent for Physicall properties, or for the Pot, yet because anciently they haue been entertained into Gardens of pleasure, their flowers hauing been in some respect, in that they haue alwaies been enterposed among the flowers of womens needle-worke, I am more willing to giue them place here then thrust them into obscurity. (249)

Through the loosely detailed but suggestively lined illustrations in the *Paradisus* (see Frontispiece), Parkinson provides a means through which the female reader can enjoy these plants not only in gardening but also in the needlework (or, as with Anne Purefoy from Chapter 2, possibly in painting) of her winter hours. In the case of the young Elizabeth Isham, these practices are often not separable.

Isham may indeed have had Parkinson specifically in her sights as the patterns provided by his large illustrations make his *Paradisus* a stronger candidate for her "book of gardening" than smaller gardening volumes by the likes of Hugh Plat, Thomas Hill, and William Lawson.[57] Along with illustrations that are useful in embroidery, moreover, intertextual evidence points to Parkinson's *Paradisus* as the transitional book in Isham's move toward medical practice; that is, the language of "delight" found in the margins of the autobiography with reference to the "seting of herbs" (marginalia fol. 19r) also appears consistently when Isham describes her needlework, and the words "delight" and "pleasure" are those used by Parkinson to describe his "earthly paradise."

This language of "delight" may point us to Parkinson's text, but it also shows that Isham may be moving away from a text that is thus focused and only partially committed to medical care. The progression of the autobiography shows a development of this language and a consequent departure from the pursuit of temporal pleasures. At first the language of pleasure reflects the medicinal aspects of meditative needlework:

> yet I found it to be ye better w^{t} me (being ye sildomer troubled) because

---

[57] Hugh Plat, *The Iewell House of Art and Nature Conteining diuers rare and profitablae inuentions, together with sundry new experimentes in the art of husbandry, distillation, and moulding* (London, 1594); Thomas Hill, *The Gardeners Labyrinth containing a discourse of the gardeners life, in the yearly trauels to be bestovved on his plot of earth, for the vse of a garden* (London, 1577); William Lawson, *A New Orchard and Garden with The Country Housewifes Garden for hearbes of common vse* (London, 1618). Lawson seems the best alternative, as roses and borage are both described as "cordial" in its pages (*Country Houewifes Garden*, 11, 12), but again, the illustrations in Parkinson make it the most likely candidate.

> [. . .] I busied & pleased my selfe w^{t} those workes of my fancy for im[m]etaing the life of [. . .] nature. as somtimes y^{e} earth & flowers, & other whiles y^{e} clouds & skie I learned in them all to Glorifie thee my God. & maker. whose workes all praise & thy Saints shall blesse thee. \psal 145.10/ & y^{e} time was y^{e} more delightfull to me because I sometimes \or daily/ read. whereby both my selfe and sister had comfort for I read in Mr Dods Booke on the commandements… (fol. 24r)

In this passage, we find that Elizabeth Isham's needlework provides a kind of preventative cure, in her "being … sildomer troubled" than her sister because of the pleasure she received through it. In this earlier episode, Isham juxtaposes the pleasures of needlework to the "delight" of reading, not romances or poetry but "Mr Dods Booke on ye com[m]andements," and the narrative gives way to praise of religious texts.

Further along in the autobiography but still before she decides to pursue herbalism, needlework's pleasures are again presented as a kind of calming medicine:

> Now hauing done the [. . .] garden flowers wch was most pleasant to me . . . I also coueted in these two som[m]ers to doe ye field flowers. & at last all y^{t} I could come by delighting much in there seuerall shaps & coullers. & though I was somthing curious to please my selfe in doing them according to ye life as much as I could. whereby it was hard. yet ye more pleasant. & I found ye more ye labour was ye more it kept me from those thoughts wch was hurtfull to mee according to ye use many times of surgions and phisitions. wch divert ye humers some other way y^{t} the may not spend themselues at one accustamed place to endanger ye health or soundnesse of ye body, but my sister delighted not to imploy her selfe this way. (fols. 25v–26r)

At the same time that it anticipates the psalmic language she will use later when turning to medicinal pursuits ("which as they are different in there shapes and coullers so are there vertues" [fol. 28r]), this passage reveals more self-censure than the previous one, which only puts needlework side by side with divine meditations. Here the use of the word "covet" to describe her needlework goals alludes to the Ten Commandments' "thou shalt not," marking it as something forbidden, and the repetition of the language of pleasure holds a more self-directed, and perhaps self-critical, syntax: the garden flowers are "most pleasant *to me*" and the desire to replicate nature was "to please my selfe." For the most part, this language of pleasure (a form of "please" or "pleasant" occurring three times) and "delight" (twice) would seem to be positive, but by the end of this passage, we find that the purpose of this delight was motivated by "surgions and phisitions," and at this point in the narrative, we know that such advice is often suspect.

Perhaps this perspective may be gained only in retrospect; however, it is important to remember that this is a crafted narrative, one that looks to create continuity and understanding in the time leading up to the time of composition. Isham's is a text that alludes to itself and wonderfully builds upon themes, and the instances in which she refers to her stitching perfectly embody that development. It is the final representation of the needlework that is most self-critical, and it is also this passage that would seem to signal a move away from these pleasures and toward more spiritual concerns. A couple of years in the narrative after she has made the resolution to learn more about medicine, the following passage appears:

> Now as Salomon made for his delight gardens & orchards. \Eccl 2.5/ so in my worke I made y^{e} shadow of these things. & I diuers times thought to make my hart reioyce in y^{e} things which I had made. wch delighted me so well when I did them. for I had devised such veriaty in little things y^{t} I might long looke & still entertaine my eyes w^{t} new obiects wch I did neere to ye life. neither had I euer seene ye like. (fol. 32v)

The author's description of her needlecraft as "shadows" undermines the pride she takes in this work, and the narrative stance, one of an older person who no longer dreams of childish things, displaces the joy in the work with introspection. Again, this is a moment when she has decided to pursue herbal knowledge, and while herbalism follows her needlework, the needlework becomes, in retrospect, a shadow of things to come. Thus the perspective of this passage as it continues is a fallen one, one that reveals a "discontent" with the "handy worke" with which she has passed her time:

> yet am I not of y^{t} opinion but there [. . .] may be as good or better handy worke of those wch haue skill by learning wch I had not. yet my owne worke many times affected me so much y^{t} I apprehended to be better then I found it to be when I (againe) looked on it: wch caused some discontent in me because it pleased me not. againe other whiles looking on it when it happened to please me I thought there was a kind of temtation in it when I looked on it too \much/ (or I found my selfe tempted to displease thee in beholding too much such vanities) Therefore I considered y^{e} vanity of these things & . . . I thought to set my mind upon better especially when these pleased me not. (fol. 32v)

This turning from "Temporall things" (fol. 32v) expressed in the movement from the "most pleasant to me" of the first passage on embroidery to the "pleased me not" and the "displease thee" found here shows us one more motivation for Isham's resolution to learn about the medicinal virtues of herbs: her spiritual path. The context provided by the sub-narrative of Isham's love for and disaffection with her embroidery helps us to better understand a marginal gloss to the moment of choosing herbalism over Latin, when she writes of the medical endeavor that she hopes "[God] wouldest be ye better pleased with me" (marginalia fol. 28r). Not only is she hoping that her God would be "better pleased" with medicine over

Latin, but she may also be indicating that her God would prefer this practice over her embroidery.

Why God would thus prefer one secular practice over another is made most clear in Isham's choice of language in the decisive passage. In considering the alternatives, Isham refers to "this way" that would benefit both her "sister and others" and thus writes of the way determined by Christ the healer (the path also followed by Mildmay and Hoby), which ultimately provides the frame for her entire work. In this autobiographical narrative and devotional meditations meant to "praise him who is ye auther of my health" (fol. 17v), from the beginning when Christ is the provider of her "soules health" (fol. 2r) to the end when she writes of the "cure" from "ye spirituall phisitian" (marginalia fol. 37r), the divine and effectual physician is the one audience she addresses directly. So while the ineffectual physicians and irreligious-but-effectual wisewomen and sorcerers give her earthly motivation for developing medical knowledge, the course is also provided in the atemporal, ever-present Christian guidance that frames the whole of her life, both as lived and as written. This perspective is gained as one considers that life as it is written in retrospect, as it develops toward the devotion that the remembrances represent.

So Elizabeth Isham's decision to own herbal knowledge in her mid-twenties is a decision bred of many motivations, histories, and circumstances. In the context of the broader society, in her role as the eldest female on a landed estate, cultural expectations legitimate the pursuit as a kind of charitable work. More immediately, her sister's health provides a direct impetus, while the history of household illness has proven that herbal cordials and cordial herbs and non-physician care are often of greatest help. The Isham familial inheritance of female medical knowledge gives Elizabeth the authoritative background, and the personal practice in needlework and gardening provide the occupational backdrop. Surrounding all is Christ's example providing "the way." This accumulation of purpose around the decision to pursue herbal knowledge demonstrates the importance of that decision in the constructions of her life history.

All being said, where is the evidence that Elizabeth Isham actually did such reading after she resolves to do so? Michelle DiMeo has found evidence that Isham was taking medical notes well into the 1640s, particularly from a translation of Giovanni da Vigo, the surgeon Mildmay read in her childhood studies, and posits that these scattered notes in the archive may constitute a "draft of . . . Isham's medical receipt book."[58] More directly in the autobiography, however, the answer lies in the margins. Aside from the great-grandmother's distillation and the "bitter Orring pilles w^t^out suger" the young Elizabeth takes to "wearme" her stomach

[58] Michelle DiMeo, "The Draft of Elizabeth Isham's Medical Receipt Book," *Constructing Elizabeth Isham*, ed. Elizabeth Clarke and Erica Longfellow, http://www2.warwick.ac.uk/fac/arts/ren/projects/isham/workshop/dimeo/ (accessed February 9, 2009).

(fol. 17v),[59] the names of herbs are found outside the main narrative. As mentioned above, it is in the margins that Elizabeth tells us about the "rosmary, roses, & borrage which [she] made conserves of" (fol. 28r) when she made the decision to pursue herbal knowledge. It is in the margins that she tells us about "the sirupt of foelfoot, and the root of elecampan in gelop" which had given her some ease when she had a cough when young and, she informs us, "since I haue made for my selfe use" (marginalia fol. 9v). In the margins we find out the names of the "herbs of hot nature" put in her mother's quilted cap, as well as into her meat and drink: rosemary, sage, marjoram, betony, and sassafras (marginalia fol. 14r). The place of herbs in the margins would seem to indicate that they were added later. Because some of the herbal cures occurred when she was a girl, as young as ten, it seems likely that she does not write these notes from deep memory but rather from present textual consultations and recent practice.[60] This insight also adds possibly

---

[59] I am convinced by the gloss provided by Michelle DiMeo for the *Constructing Elizabeth Isham* project that these are "bitter orange peels."

[60] I would like to hypothesize here, in the margins of this analysis, that the herbal she reads while writing the marginalia is John Parkinson's *Theatrum Botanicum* (page numbers below are taken from that text). My hypothesis stems from the evidence provided in the 1648 book inventory; namely, "An Herball," rather than a generic title, I propose, refers to *Theatrum*'s subtitle, "an herball of a large extent." My speculation goes along with my other proposal that for the "book of gardening," the book inventoried after the herbal, we are to consider the *Paradisus*, which Parkinson saw as volume one of the two-volume series. My proposition is also rooted in the shared language between Isham's *Remembrances* and Parkinson's text. It is not simply that Parkinson recommends "the freshe roots of Elecampane" (655) and a "Syrup made" of "the fresh leaues or juyce" of foalfoot (1220) to "helpe the cough" (655) or that *Theatrum* also lists all of the "herbs of hot nature" from the mother's treatment as hot; these qualities may be found in other works. It is the particular language of cordials and conserves, from the narrative in general but pointedly in the decision to read about herbs—the conserves of rosemary, rose, and borage that were "cordial for her"—that signifies the relationship between texts. Importantly, this language is not found in Gerard, the most likely alternative (and his is pointedly entitled "*The* Herball"), but is everywhere in both of Parkinson's texts. For example, "the flowers and the conserve made of [rosemary]" is "singular good to comfort the heart" (77), and "the dry conserve which is called Sugar of Roses is a very good Cordiall to strengthen the heart and spirits" (1022). Most convincing is *Theatrum*'s entry on borage, which begins by apologizing for only a slight discussion of borage's important medical benefits in his previous volume and continues with the description of this virtue: "the Conserue made of the flowers, or the flowers candid [*sic*] are helping also in all those causes, but are chiefely used as a Cordiall, and good for those that have beene long sicke and feeble or in a Consumption, to comfort the heart and spirits, and thereby good for those that are troubled with often swounings or passions of the heart" (768). The wording here almost seems to describe the sister whose brittle bones and "vitall parts" (fol. 30v) caused her misery and kept her in bed throughout her youth, whose disposition was often despairing in her illness and only joyous in considering death, and whose young life ended when Elizabeth, her older sister, was only twenty-seven.

another textual dimension to the autobiography as it becomes a means of study; that is, in the marginalia, Isham conceivably could return to scenes of illness to diagnose and remedy in retrospect what had ailed herself and her loved ones. This possible reading recognizes that through the autobiography, Elizabeth Isham bears witness to the deaths of not only a beloved grandmother, mother, and sister, but also, in the last pages, a sister-in-law and nephew, and posits that, while she can no longer care for them and watch by their bedside, she can minister to and in their memory. In capturing herbal reading in the margins of her life narrative, she memorializes her family at the same time that she fulfills one life decision justified in the text.

Isham's purposefulness in retrospect differs from the use of the herbal text represented by Hoby and Mildmay in their narratives, as Hoby provides a series of substitutions and variances in her daily accounting and Mildmay frames her educational and practical accretion as the building of her legacy. Also, Isham's development of her practice against licensed medical authority rather than in collaboration with that authority in the manner of Hoby and Mildmay gives us an alternative view of the role the herbal plays in a woman's medical practice. In their different generic purposes and their contrasting relationships with the licensed physician, the examples of Mildmay, Hoby, and Isham open for us the variety of meanings available through the representation of one kind of text, even when that text is not literary. And for this reason, I want to propose that the category of "the literary" may limit the intertextual potentials that we attribute to women's texts. Elizabeth Isham's decision not to learn Latin should not be viewed as a gender limitation but rather a choice with deep sociological significance; her decision to pursue herbal knowledge does not handicap her writing but rather determines the ways meaning may be formed within it. Grace Mildmay's extensive medical notebooks may seem cryptic to us now, but the processes of experimentation and annotation show how the writing mind may work and how one may revise, enumerate, and expand as one depicts one's life. Lady Hoby may never have read Edmund Spenser, but she reads a variety of books with various uses and intents and engages a wide community through her reading. For those of us who have passed our language exams, have taught Virgil and Spenser, and have gained the other "doctor" title, the reading of the herbal may seem utilitarian and thus limited in significance. But when we consider the context of the life and how the herbal knowledge is claimed in that life, the herbal gains critical importance through the social dimensions it highlights in the text being written.

Thus this larger study ends with a consideration of a poetic text, Isabella Whitney's *Sweet Nosgay*. As of yet, *Sweet Nosgay*'s intertextuality has mainly been thought of with regard to other literary texts and other works by women.[61]

---

[61] Previous intertextual analysis of Isabella Whitney's poetry include: Richard Panofsky, ed., The Floures of Philosophie *(1572) by Sir Hugh Plat and* A Sweet Nosgay *(1573) and* The Copy of a Letter *(1567) by Isabella Whitney* (Delmar, New York: Scholars' Facsimiles and Reprints, 1982); Ann Rosalind Jones, *The Currency of Eros*: *Women's Love*

In considering Whitney's *Nosgay* as an herbal text, this study asks us to consider alternative intertextual potentials for the volume. In looking for these potentials, we must first consider the differences of the *Nosgay* volume and of the author's position as she represents it. A poor woman lacking employment in London, Whitney wrote *Nosgay* not simply to circulate among family members and closest counselors, but rather to appear in print; that the volume appears in octavo proves to be an essential clue in assessing its intertextuality. In considering *Nosgay* with regard to the author's socio-economic and geographic location and the book's size and affordability, this study points to the author's complicated relationship to licensed medical authority and thus further develops our appreciation of the social satire found throughout Whitney's herbal text.

Lyric in Europe, 1540–1620 (Bloomington: Indiana University Press, 1990), 37–52; Wendy Wall, *The Imprint of Gender: Authorship and Publication in the English Renaissance* (Ithaca: Cornell University Press, 1993), 283–310; Ilona Bell, *Elizabethan Women and the Poetry of Courtship* (Cambridge: Cambridge University Press, 1998), 13–25; Mary Ellen Lamb, "Isabella Whitney and the Travails of Service" (paper presented at the meeting of the Renaissance Society of America, Miami, Florida, March 24, 2007).

Chapter 4
Isabella Whitney's Herbs: Print Medical Texts and London Satire

Anyone who reads Isabella Whitney's 1573 collection of poems faces a most vivid structural metaphor for the volume: as the poet presents it in her address to the reader, the collection is a "sweet nosgay" that will protect its readership from a plague-like disease of the mind. This "posye" is constituted not only by the poeticization of selected aphorisms from Hugh Plat's *The floures of philosophie, with the pleasures of poetrie annexed to them* (1572) called "flowers,"[1] but also by the poems of advice and good will written to family and friends that follow these short verses. She refers to her poems throughout the address to the reader as "my Nosegay" (sig. A7v) and "vertuous Flowers" (sig. A4v). That the flowers are "vertuous" points directly to their medicinal virtues; the poet tells her reader that, as Plat's text served as her "defence" "[i]n stynking streets or lothsome Lanes" (A6v) of London, she presents the poems for the reader's "health, not for [his/her] eye" (sig. A7r). She does so because she "did safety finde" (sig. A7r) in Plat, and she offers her poetry to her reader as an act of "good wyll" (sig. A7r). The virtues of Isabella Whitney's herbs, some of which are picked from Plat's "ground" (sig. A7v) or "Plot" (sig. A8r), therefore, are that they protect the reader from the moral contagions in the metaphoric "aire" (sig. A5r) of London through their lyrical sweet scent. That the metaphor is meant to apply to the whole volume and not just the verses derived from Plat is clear when she uses the word "prescribed" to describe the "order" (sig. C7v) she provides for her younger sisters to "prevent" a moral "infect[ion]" (sig. C8r) while they are serving-maids in London. Whitney gives her sisters advice ratified through her experience in service (the poet having lost her position for some not fully disclosed reason)[2] and, as with Plat's sentiments, offers her prescription because it has worked for her, giving her readership an "approved"

---

1 See Richard J. Panofsky, ed., The Floures of Philosophie *by Sir Hugh Plat and* A Sweet Nosgay *(1573) and* The Copy of a Letter *(1567) by Isabella Whitney* (Delmar, New York: Scholars' Facsimiles and Reprints, 1982). Edition used in this analysis is Isabella Whitney, *A Sweet Nosgay* (London: 1573), *Renaissance Women Online*, September, 1999, Women Writers Project, Brown University, http://textbase.wwp.brown.edu/WWO/php/rAll.php?doc=whitney.nosegay.html&num=00280 (accessed February 28, 2009). Citations included in the text.

2 Anne Rosalind Jones argues for "defamation" by "enemies" in "Maidservants of London: Sisterhoods of Kinship and Labor," in *Maids and Mistresses, Cousins and Queens: Women Alliances in Early Modern England*, ed. Susan Frye and Karen Robertson (New

medicine. While many critics have made the connection to women's domestic practice of medicine,[3] this chapter attempts to demonstrate how the connection to household practice may be made too readily and conclusively, closing off a very suggestive set of signifiers. Going beyond this connection to the domestic, my analysis here sets out to delineate the complex economics of authorial herbalism through the metaphors and intertextuality of Isabella Whitney's *Sweet Nosgay*.

Whitney never names the herbs that constitute her remedy. Such literal "nose-herbs"—as they are called by Lafeu in Act V, scene 5 of *All's Well That Ends Well*—are many, not only including Lavatch's sweet marjoram and rue, but also lilies, violets, and rosemary, among others.[4] The "flowers" taken from Plat are only numbered, never named, importantly leaving them in the realm of metaphor. This metaphorization does not simply abstract Whitney's intent and allude to a generalizable medicine in a widely variable context, however; rather, in line with my argument throughout this study, Whitney's insistence on comparing her poems to effective medicinal plants has very particular social ramifications. The poet presents this posy to a specific audience, one that lives in London where the plague threatens to decimate the populace and where medical care is regulated (however "loosely") by the College of Physicians; as a result, in the city, physician care could be in high demand and very expensive, thus making poorer individuals dependent on "irregular" practitioners.[5] So through this frame of reference, Whitney taps

York: Oxford University Press, 1999), 24. There is also the implication that her ill health may have been a contributing factor.

[3] Kim Walker, *Women Writers of the English Renaissance* (New York: Twayne Publishers, 1996), 161; Jane Donawerth, "Women's Poetry and the Tudor–Stuart System of Gift Exchange," in *Women, Writing, and the Reproduction of Culture in Tudor and Stuart Britain*, ed. Mary E. Burke, Jane Donawerth, Linda L. Dove, and Karen Nelson (New York: Syracuse University Press, 2000), 14–15; Wendy Wall, "Authorship and the Material Conditions of Writing," in *The Cambridge Companion to English Literature, 1500–1600*, ed. Arthur F. Kinney (Cambridge: Cambridge University Press, 2000), 75; Patricia Phillippy, "The Maid's Lawful Liberty: Service, the Household, and 'Mother B' in Isabella Whitney's *A Sweet Nosegay*," *Modern Philology* 95.4 (1998): 458–62; Patricia Brace, "Isabella Whitney, *A Sweet Nosegay*," in *A Companion to Early Modern Women's Writing*, ed. Anita Pacheco (Oxford: Blackwell Publishing, 2002), 97–109; Lynette McGrath, *Subjectivity and Women's Poetry in Early Modern England* (Aldershot, Hampshire: Ashgate Publishing, 2002), 151; Laurie Ellinghausen, "Literary Property and the Single Woman in Isabella Whitney's *A Sweet Nosegay*," *Studies in English Literature* 45.1 (Winter 2005): 6–7. Brace does move Whitney's work into the "literary marketplace" but does not explore the medicinal aspects of the plants in this economic context, "Isabella Whitney," 99.

[4] William Shakespeare, *All's Well That Ends Well*, in *The Norton Shakespeare*, ed. Stephen Greenblatt et al. (New York: W. W. Norton, 1997), 4.5.16.

[5] On London's "loose regulation" of its medical market, see Deborah Harkness, *The Jewel House: Elizabethan London and the Scientific Revolution* (New Haven, Connecticut: Yale University Press, 2007), 65. See Margaret Pelling (with Frances White), *Medical Conflicts in Early Modern London: Patronage, Physicians, and Irregular Practitioners,*

into the *pathos* of London fears about and memories of disease; that is, through evoking the experience of illness, the writer provides an emotional background for her argument.[6] In providing an affordable (if figurative) medicine to a general audience, she establishes the *ethos* of her work in its healing capacity (a precursor, perhaps, to the "ethos of care" that Katharine Gillespie sees in seventeenth-century dissent writings by Elizabeth Poole and Mary Cary),[7] and, as we will see, this ethical stance has much to do with the economic disparities of the London market. At the same time that her metaphor of the nosegay raises the specters of deadly contagion and expensive medicine for the rhetorical ends of her work, in keeping her herbs figurative, Whitney is also immune from the strictures imposed by the College. She is immune even though she enters its jurisdiction. Thus the metaphor works on two levels: through the frame of herbal preventative, the poet introduces an economic critique maintained throughout the *Nosgay* volume, and through metaphorization, she shields that critique from any real-world censure.

In this way, Whitney's metaphoric herbs are not simply a literary manifestation of the gentlewomen's practice witnessed in Mildmay, Hoby, and Isham. As we have seen, even the gentlewomen's herbal readings represent different relationships to physicians, and in a similar manner Whitney's herbalism signifies a particular relationship to licensed medical authorities. Applying the language of Roger Chartier, her "contrasted use" of the medical knowledge in front of her is dependent on the specificities of her context,[8] and these in turn distinguish hers from the women's writings examined in the third chapter. Unlike the writers Mildmay and Hoby, Whitney's persona is that of a single woman. Unlike Elizabeth Isham, she has no source of income and is "very weake in Purse" (sig. E3r). Unlike all three as well, she does not simply visit or hear reports of London; at the beginning of the collection, she has been living in its heart. She is a woman of the city. Unlike the works written in the countryside, moreover, which were written mainly for their authors' own edification and for that of their family members and immediate friends, *Sweet Nosgay* appears in print in an affordable octavo volume and is the second public work Whitney has had set to the press, following *The Copy of a Letter* (1567). These factors—Whitney's economic and marital status, the

1550–1640 (Oxford: Clarendon Press, 2003); Pelling discusses the different kinds of "irregular practitioners" taken before the College.

6 In this statement, my work reveals its relationship to that of Raymond A. Anselment, whose consideration of literature in the context of the extensive illnesses in the early modern period turns to the rhetoric of counsel and consolation, *The Realms of Apollo: Literature and Healing in Seventeenth-Century England* (Newark: University of Delaware Press, 1995).

7 Katharine Gillespie, *Domesticity and Dissent in the Seventeenth Century: English Women Writers and the Public Sphere* (Cambridge: Cambridge University Press, 2004), 53.

8 Roger Chartier, *Cultural History: Between Practices and Representations*, trans. Lydia G. Cochrane (Ithaca, New York: Cornell University Press, 1988), 13.

author's location in London, and the work's appearance in print—all contribute to the specificity of her herbalism and with it the poet's relationship to medical authority.

In the past two decades, many critics have been articulating Whitney's position "as a poor, single woman who explicitly claims to write for money,"[9] and my intent here is to consider the importance of herbalism in this articulation. Laurie Ellinghausen's challenge for us to consider "the meaning of 'textual communities'" to "writers who looked to anonymous consumers as their primary source of monetary support" has particularly interesting ramifications when that "support" is constructed as the purchase of herbs.[10] Patricia Phillippy and Anne Rosalind Jones differently interpret Whitney's self-presentation as a former maidservant (or a female servant of slightly higher status) in the context of the pamphlet *A Letter sent by the Maydens of London* (1567).[11] Their analyses with regard to this pamphlet, which was written in defense of aspersions made against serving-maids, help us in considering the specificities of Whitney's constructed position, and I would like to add to their observations Fiona McNeill's recent discussion of poor women's "making shift," turning to alternative trades, when they would lose employment in a household and were cast into the streets of London without a means of income.[12] When turning to the herbal frame of the volume, these previous considerations of the *Nosgay* persona's status fall back on practice found within the household rather than interrogating the specific London milieu, but if we revise these observations with the idea that the poet has to "make shift" in losing her position, we see that she does so on a literal level through her writing and on a figurative level by selling an herbal preventative against a dis-eased mind. While some may recognize the "labor" of the poet's gathering the herbs, no one has yet considered the implications of the poet's *selling* herbs (however metaphoric) to a London audience. As Whitney's text as well as others to be considered in this chapter let us know, in the early modern period, London was a city filled with both physical and metaphysical disease, and selling herbs has a particular import in such a context.

In terms of the helpful structural analysis performed by Sara Jayne Steen, the importance of London is made readily apparent in the volume's first and fourth sections, but can be felt throughout the text.[13] While the second section, subtitled "A sweet Nosgay, Or pleasant Posye: contayning a hundred and ten Phylosophicall

[9] Ellinghausen, "Literary Property and the Single Woman," 1.

[10] Ellinghausen, "Literary Property and the Single Woman," 20.

[11] Phillippy, "Maid's Lawful Liberty;" Jones, "Maidservants of London."

[12] Fiona McNeill, *Poor Women in Shakespeare* (Cambridge: Cambridge University Press, 2007), 13.

[13] Sara Jayne Steen, "Contextual Materials for *A Sweet Nosgay*," Introductions to Works, *Renaissance Women Online*, September 1999, Women Writers Project, Brown University, http://textbase.wwp.brown.edu/WWO/php/rInt.php?doc=rInt.00280.html&LT (accessed March 2, 2009).

Flowers, &c" (sig. B2r), the versified passages from Plat's *Floures of philosophie* with the short poem "A soveraigne receypt" and the envoy "A farewell to the Reader" (sig. C5r), is ostensibly the center, the flowers themselves take up less than half of the entire *Nosgay* volume. Again, central to our understanding of *Nosgay* is the function of the flowers, to protect the reader from a plague-like disease, which has particular resonance for a London readership in 1573. In the London context, the thirteen "familier [verse] Epistles and friendly Letters by the Auctor" (sig. C6r) addressed to family and friends—including the moral preventative prescription to her younger sisters—that comprise the third section of the volume function to reveal her social network and to emphasize her isolation within the city.[14] The prefatory first section, an extensive prose dedicatory letter to George Mainwaring and an address from "The Auctor to the Reader" (sig.A5r) and the last—a kind of "farewell" for the whole volume—her "Wyll and Testament" to the city of London, are arguably the most original and poetical of the sections and explicitly frame the work as written from within London. From the opening address the author walks its "stynking streetes" on her "businesse" (A6v) and, in the end, finds it too expensive for her to stay within its vicinity. These explicit references to the city thus color the rest of volume. In the center of the action and the danger (particularly in the form of the plague), Whitney writes to her close relations and perceives the need for protective medicines; as a result, she sends a figurative nosegay against foul-smelling mental contagion not only to her loved ones but to the unknown reader as well.

As London was the center of the book trade in early modern England, it makes sense that the two contexts of print and the city have related ramifications. Within the context of London, we encounter the book market, an arena represented by Whitney herself in the "Bookebinders stall" (sig. E7r) of "Wyll and Testament," and we find ourselves within the same geographic area as the College of Physicians. Whereas manuscript texts written for a limited audience are less likely to fall under the College's regulation, a small print text—which would have been more widely affordable than larger texts—circulating in London existed within a setting in which medical practice was most policed, i.e., in a context in which a practitioner looking to make money would ostensibly have needed a license. Whitney created the persona of a woman pursuing an income by giving her London readers medicinal herbs, and in doing so raised the specter of possible censure. Again, after 1542 unlicensed individuals could practice only if they did not charge a fee. Print thus changes the context of herbal practice from the household environment to that of the London market, and in doing so it must circumvent any regulations she may have been perceived to transgress. It is the metaphorization of her herbs

---

[14] For extended discussions of this isolation, see Walker, *Women Writers*, 156–62, and Ellinghausen, "Literary Property and the Single Woman," 8. Phillippy adds that this isolation is in part due to the migratory experience of serving-maids in the period, "Maid's Lawful Liberty," 452–53.

that allows for this circumvention, or, put another way, she transgresses, yet only metaphorically.

Appearing in print also places Whitney's work in the company of other books. Other print texts from Whitney's decade certainly draw upon medicinal metaphors in making scriptural/moral arguments, even going so far as to call their works "nosegays."[15] Susan Felch has discussed the "authorial medicine" of Ann Lock in delivering John Calvin's sermons, and religious authors from our own William Turner to John Knox have all drawn on the rhetorical and allusive potentials of remedy as metaphor.[16] While later authors such as Anne Wheathill engaged these devotional texts directly, adding layers to their volumes, it is my contention that Whitney's source texts are much more literal and thus differently polemical;[17] in making her moral argument, Whitney articulates parallels between her writing and that of authors of print medical texts, not other metaphorical texts. If we consider *Nosgay* within the context of print herbal texts, we can begin to see how it fits within a larger social critique about economic inaccessibility of licensed medical care and how satire is a central vein of the entire volume, not just its last section. In my emphasis on economics, my reading bows to Elaine Beilin and with her, Patricia Brace, both of whom have approached Whitney's "Wyll and Testament" "along class lines," considering the economic disparities within that poem's London and the poet's satirical stance against it.[18] In essence, I would like to look at how such an approach may be applied to the entire volume and how the lens of

---

15 Thomas Becon, *A pleasante newe Nosegaye* (London, 1542); Gabriel Meurier, *The Nosegay of Morall Philosophie*, trans. Thomas Crew (London, 1580).

16 Susan Felch, "Ann Lock's Authorial Medicine," *Reformation* 2 (1997): 7–38. William Turner, *A new booke of spirituall Physik for dyuerse diseases of the nobilite and gentlemen of Englande* (Rome, 1555); John Knox, *A fort for the afflicted: VVherein are ministred many notable & excellent remedies against the stormes of tribulation* (London, 1580), first written in 1554. See also any number of works in Thomas Becon, *The Worckes of Thomas Becon* (London, 1560–1564); the anonymous text, *A godly and holsom preseruatyue against disperacion at al times necessarye for the soule* (London, 1551); and Paul Bush, *Certayne Gostly Medycynes to be Used to Eschew the Plage of Pestilence* (London, 1531), among others. For a discussion of this branch of vernacular physic, see Paul Slack, "Mirrors of Health and Treasures of Poor Men: The Uses of Vernacular Medical Literature of Tudor England," in *Health, Medicine, and Mortality in the Sixteenth Century*, ed. Charles Webster (Cambridge: Cambridge University Press, 1979), 254–56.

17 Anne Wheathill, *A handfull of holesome (though homelie) hearbs, gathered out of the goodlie garden of Gods most holie word* (London, 1584).

18 Elaine Beilin, *Redeeming Eve: Women Writers of the English Renaissance* (Princeton: Princeton University Press, 1987), 99; Patricia Brace, "Teaching Class: Whitney's 'Wyll and Testament' and Nashe's 'Litany in Time of Plague,'" in *Teaching Tudor and Stuart Women Writers*, ed. Susanne Woods and Margaret Hannay (New York: The Modern Language Assocation, 2000), 279–82. See also Wendy Wall's discussion of "Wyll" in *The Imprint of Gender: Authorship and Publication in the English Renaissance* (Ithaca, New York: Cornell University Press, 1993), 283–31.

medical texts from the period surrounding Whitney's publication can allow us to discern the terms of Whitney's critique. In general, I mean to keep the context of economic disparities in health care at the center of our consideration of Whitney's medical metaphors.

In the light of economic inequities, Whitney's relationship to medical authority seems in no way unproblematic, and tensions do arise in the poetry as a result of her status and her geographic position. At the beginning of the volume we find that the poet is "harvestlesse" and "servicelesse" (sig. A5v), without household and without employment (as Phillippy points out in both country [harvest] and city [service]);[19] thus it would be a mistake to position her with other gentlewomen who practice medicine among the poor because the story the poet tells from the outset is one about the need for assistance, not the assistance of the needy. Her clientele are paying customers—albeit for metaphoric herbs—and her work circulates in the backyard of the College. Caught "beyond the . . . confines of the home"[20] and positioning herself as a provider of public remedy within London, the poet-as-practitioner must negotiate the city's strictures on lay medical practice. Gentlewomen such as Hoby and Mildmay have no such negotiations to perform.

There are reasons, however, why previous critics have wanted to place Whitney's metaphoric herbalism within the context of domestic practice. One of these is the "gifts" or "presents" she makes of the herbs to her friend and patron George Mainwaring, her brother Geoffrey Whitney (and with him her former employer), and her sister Anne Baron. In the familiar letters to siblings above her in status, she metonymically refers at once to the individual poem and the general volume in terms of simplicity; to Anne she writes, "good Sister take . . . / These simple lynes that come from mee" (sig. D1v), and to Geoffrey, "Receave of me, and eke accept, / a simple token" (sig. C6v). In the second instance, "the simple token," the *Nosgay*, is at once for two individuals above her, her brother and the "vertuous Lady" to whom Isabella asks him to bring the "present," the woman whose employ she recently had left behind. These instances in the letters to her siblings echo the moments in which Whitney uses the word "simple" in the dedicatory epistle to George Mainwaring.[21] In that letter she refers to "this simple Nosegaye" (sig. A4r) and, through the parable of the poor man who brings water in his hands to the "Persian Prince," a "Simple Guift" (sig. A4v). In all four instances, "simple" characterizes the individual epistle as representative of the entire collection of verses while at the same time it implicitly points to the poor woman behind the poetry; that is, the multiple meanings of "simple" create a hierarchic tension in the relationship between the reader, who receives healing advice but also has economic power, and the author, who offers a wholesome product but is economically susceptible.

---

19 Phillippy, "Maid's Lawful Liberty," 444.

20 Phillippy, "Maid's Lawful Liberty," 462.

21 Noted in Walker, *Women Writers*, 159.

On one level, "simple" puns on the central conceit of the work, that the volume is preventative medicine for the benefit of the reader. Donawerth opens the door to this reading when she writes "Whitney begins and ends [the] section of maxims in *Nosgay* by presenting her poems as herbal medicine, the kind of gift frequently made and exchanged by women."[22] It thus follows that many of the direct references to gifts in the poem are framed herbally, for "simple," as we have seen throughout this study, means a medicine of a pure ingredient. In this way, Whitney identifies *Nosgay* as a gift made of simples, or individual herbs, and she indicates to her sister, brother, former employer, and patron that she is attending to their health as many women in the period shared their medicine with persons of their acquaintance. In giving members of her circle a medicinal nosegay, Whitney frames her poetic volume as one of charitable or domestic work, meant to preserve their health and through them in her "good will" that of others they may know. We see such examples of this domestic work in letters written by Lady Brilliana Harley and the gentlewoman Maria Thynne, who respectively send son and husband residing in London remedies for the plague when they hear that the sickness has surfaced.[23] Again, the difference here is that the poet is not safe in the countryside overseeing a household in her husband's absence; on the contrary, single and unemployed, she resides in London, and, in need of money, she is selling her remedy to an unknown audience.

So, on another level, through the word "simple," Whitney points to differences in status and education between herself and the more privileged members of her readership. "Simple" can mean uneducated and poor (a wonderful source of comedy when the character Simple hides in the doctor's closet in *The Merry Wives of Windsor)*—most always, it seems, relative to a more elite party—and it is through these connotations that Whitney would seem to be invoking the modesty topos discussed by Boyd Berry.[24] In this regard, she structures an audience upon whom she is dependent for money (the former employer and the patron) and below whom she otherwise exists on the social scale (her married sister and her brother). These gifts, therefore, are not exchanged as between gentlewomen of equal economic capacities, and Whitney's differentiated status distinguishes her practice from that of previously discussed gentlewomen practitioners. In other

---

22 Donawerth, "Women's Poetry and the Tudor–Stuart System of Gift Exchange," 14.

23 The letter in which Lady Harley sends Ned a piece of angelica can be found in *Letters of the Lady Brilliana Harley*, Brilliana Harley, *Letters of the Lady Brilliana Harley, Wife of Sir Robert Harley, of Brampton Bryan, Knight of Bath*, ed. and intro., Thomas Taylor Lewis, A.M., vicar of Bridstow, Herefordshire (London: Camden Society, 1854, 129. Maria Thynne, "Letters," in *Lay by Your Needles Ladies, Take the Pen: Writing Women in England, 1500–1700*, ed. Suzanne Trill, Kate Chedgzoy, and Melanie Osborne (London: St. Martin's Press, 1997), 77.

24 Boyd Berry, "'We are not all alyke nor of complexion one': Truism and Isabella Whitney's Multiple Readers," *Renaissance Papers* (2000): 17.

interactions with her audience, for example in the address to the reader, even though Whitney frames her poem as an act of "good wyll," she brings it into the system of mercantile exchange, thus transforming any household or charitable signifiers. Again, in this change in domestic signifiers, Whitney's work carries the potential of a metaphoric transgression. Whitney uses medical metaphors with a sense of her audience that is not simply the familial or the known. As both Phillippy and Ellinghausen point out, the inclusion of the letters to the family members emphasizes the physical or metaphysical separation of the poet from her most immediate circle, i.e., from what would otherwise be her household.[25] This separation in turn subjects her to an undetermined audience. In light of this indeterminacy, she addresses, in Berry's phrase, "multiple readers" and negotiates the public forum with her herbal language.

The poet's difference in status and susceptibility to public censure is most readily felt in the specter of witchcraft that Whitney invokes in the closing of her address to the reader. Whereas Elizabeth Isham assures her divine audience that she and her family never directly interacted with practitioners who "used inderict meanes,"[26] the *Nosgay* poet, as a woman of few means and offering herbal remedies to the reading public, has different worries. As Margaret Pelling, William Kerwin, Bella Mirabella, and others have discussed, if a woman practiced medicine in the streets of London, she was no longer taking part in the "Renaissance housewife's prescribed task of attending to bodily ailments" described by Wendy Wall;[27] she was playing with something much more dangerous and ultimately prohibited.[28] One need only recall John Gerard's virulent decree against "witches, charmers, & such like couseners that regarde more to get money, then to helpe for charitie"[29] to see witchcraft's associations with mercantile herbal practice by women. Under the witchcraft statutes of 1542, renewed by Elizabeth I in 1563 after a brief hiatus under Edward VI and Mary, witch trials such as those in Essex throughout the 1560s and 1570s (and well into the 1580s) were known in the London streets through pamphlets and public executions.[30] Alongside the witchcraft statutes,

---

25 Phillippy, "Maid's Lawful Liberty," 462, and Ellinghausen, "Literary Property and the Single Woman," 8.

26 Elizabeth Isham, "Autobiography, ca. 1640s," Robert H. Taylor Collection, Princeton University Library, RTC01 no. 62, fol. 18v.

27 Wall, "Authorship and the Material Conditions of Writing," 75.

28 Pelling, *Medical Conflicts in Early Modern London*; William Kerwin, *Beyond the Body: The Boundaries of Medicine and English Renaissance Drama* (Amherst: University of Massachusetts Press, 2005); Bella Mirabella, "'Quacking Delilahs': Female Mountebanks in Early Modern England and Italy," in *Women Players in England, 1500–1650: Beyond the All-Male Stage*, ed. Pamela Allen Brown and Peter Parolin (Burlington, Vermont: Ashgate Publishing, 2005), 89–105.

29 John Gerard, *The Herball or Generall Historie of Plantes* (London, 1597), 288.

30 For example, see, "The Confessions of the Chelmsford Witches: England [1566]," in *Witchcraft in Europe, 400–1700: A Documentary History*, ed. Alan Charles Kors and

women, although not as systematically as men, were regularly brought in front of the College of Physicians for practicing without a license.[31] Certainly, censure of female practice existed elsewhere through the ecclesiastical courts, but these state-run regulations, when combined with the paranoia brought about by the 1563 plague (the same year that the witchcraft statutes were renewed), which killed a reported 20,000 people in London, made one's role as a female London practitioner at best needed, at worst hangable.[32] By extension, Whitney's conceit that she delivers a helpful medicine to her London readership is tinged with the presence of this metaphoric danger as she articulates in these memorable prefatory lines from her address:

> Wherfore, if thou it hap to weare
> and feele thy selfe much worse:
> Promote mee for no Sorceresse,
> nor doe mée ban or curse. (sig. A8r)

As these lines clearly assert and Deborah Harkness's analysis of the historical records supports, "happy clients were any practitioner's best defense."[33] In the worst instance, she could be put on trial as a witch, and if things went wrong, she could be publicly ostracized or "banned," possibly a reference to censure by the College. The poet recognizes that she has made herself vulnerable by offering a public remedy for pay and that she could be blamed for another's illness. In line with Kerwin's understanding of the female practitioner's position as a "multidimensional Medea" in early modern London and theater, Whitney's self-positioning here acknowledges her own outlier status as a practitioner.[34] This is a position that is pointedly removed from the household.

This outlier position when aligned with her lower economic status means that the poet's relationship to the expensive physician is minimal, occurring only in the direst circumstances, and, at times, even oppositional, being open to censure from the physician. Unlike Mildmay, Hoby, and Isham, who consult or encounter physicians regularly, Whitney tells her reader that she or he should see "Sir *Medicus* with [his] stronger Earbes" (sig. A7v) only if his or her "mind" is already

---

Edward Peters, 2nd ed., rev. Edward Peters (Philadelphia: University of Pennsylvania Press, 2001), 302–308. Alan MacFarlane has commented on the trials in this region extensively, *Witchcraft in Tudor and Stuart England: A Regional and Comparative Study* (New York: Harper and Row Publishers, 1970).

[31] A lengthy discussion of these cases can be found in Pelling's chapter, "Gendered Compromises: The Female Practitioner and her Connections," *Medical Conflicts in Early Modern London*, 189–224.

[32] Leslie A. Clarkson, *Death, Disease, and Famine in Pre-Industrial England* (New York: St. Martin's Press, 1975), 66.

[33] Harkness, *The Jewel House*, 74.

[34] Kerwin, *Beyond the Body*, 68.

"infected" and her herbs will not "prevayle" (sig. A7r). Thus the poet's medicine, though it may be subject to a "ban" by him (sig. A8r), precedes the need for the physician's care and exists outside any direct exchange with medical authority as represented by that physician. Importantly, in preceding him, she proposes to give her readership a way of avoiding him and his fee.

Ultimately, Whitney's presence in this study reminds us of the economics of medical care in early modern London. Whereas the gentlewomen examined in the previous chapters interacted with physicians with seeming ease and their charitable practice alleviated the needs of the poor, Whitney's poetic position as a woman otherwise without income who extends a kind of herbal medicine to a paying London public provides a different perspective on the subject. That is, as Christopher Hill and others have shown us, one of the consequences of medical regulation in and around London in the early modern period was higher costs for such licensed medical care.[35] Evidence of both the problem and the remedy for it can be found in many of the paratextual elements from print medical texts from the 1560s and 1570s, as these volumes claimed that the ability to self-administer or a general practice outside of licensure could help alleviate these costs. In an example we have already seen in Chapter 1, Henry Lyte's address to his herbal's reader, the author gives this reason for publication:

> that euen the meanest of my Countriemen (whose skill is not so profounde that they can fetche this knowledge out of strange tongues, nor their habilitie so wealthy, as to entertaine a learned Phisition) may yet in time of their necessitie, haue some helpes in their owne, or their neighbours fieldes and gardens at home.[36]

Even though his herbal was expensive relative to smaller books, Lyte proposes that it would still be cost effective for the purchaser when compared to the services of the physician. Titles of smaller and more affordable volumes such as *The Poor mans Ievvel* (1578) and *The Treasure of poore men* (1560) speak directly to the minor costs of purchasing a book against consulting with a licensed individual, and the often republished *The Myrrour or Glass of Healthe* by Thomas Moulton (2nd ed., 1566) verbalizes the author's "compassion" for "the poore people," who are "distroied euery daye therby for defaute of helpe."[37] Other texts yet again

---

35 Christopher Hill, "The Medical Profession and Its Radical Critics," in *Change and Continuity in Seventeenth-Century England* (Cambridge, Massachusetts: Harvard University Press, 1975), 157–77.

36 Henry Lyte, "To the friendly and indifferent Reader," from his translation of Rembert Dodoens's *A Nievve Herball, or Historie of Plantes* (London, 1578), sig.*3r.

37 Thomas Brasbridge, *The Poore Mans Ievvel, that is to say, A Treatise of the Pestilence Unto the which is Annexed a declaration of the vertues of the hearbs Carduus Benedictus and Angelica* (London, 1578); Anonymous, *Here Begynneth a Good Booke of Medecines Called the Treasure of poore men* (London, 1560?); Thomas Moulton, *The*

exhibit a more direct censure of "them that are of better learninge" who would have medicine kept "secret for lucre of the few."[38] The translator of Jean Goeurot's *Regiment of lyfe* (1567) asks,

> How long wolde they haue the people ignorant? why grutche they phisicke to come forth in Englishe? would they haue no man knowe but onely they? Or what make they them selues? Marcha[n]tes of our liues & deathes, that wee shuld bie our health onely of them, and at their prices, no good phisicion is of that minde.[39]

The image of the good physician, who provides remedy for little or no cost to the much neglected poor, against that of the implicitly bad physician, who would benefit from the hoarding of knowledge and power, accounts for the popularity of print texts of all sizes that provided knowledge in herbal and general medicine. It is this context into which I now would like to bring the question of how Isabella Whitney's herbs communicate a vexed relationship to licensed medical authority.

Whitney's Texts

Whitney presents her volume as a text engaged with other texts. Her persona calls upon various kinds of reading such as scripture, histories, and the classics as well as her source text, Hugh Plat's *Floures*, and in this way makes hers a volume that is highly intertextual. Most immediately, Ann Rosalind Jones and Lynette McGrath have taken the overt presence of Ovid's *Heroides* in Whitney's early *A Copy of a Letter* and applied the letter of complaint to *Nosgay*, and in her current project, Mary Ellen Lamb, following Richard Panofsky, analyzes this intertextuality at play in the history of Senecan *sententiae* as represented by Plat.[40] Through the avenues of gender, Wendy Wall, in her early work, explores the interplay between Whitney's "Wyll" and print pamphlets of mother's advice written as wills as well as "Ovidian complaint" and "city satire."[41] Remembering the libraries of Anne

---

Myrrour or Glass of Healthe (London, [1566]), n.p. The quote can be found on the first page after the table of contents.

38 Thomas Phaire, "Preface to the Reader," in Jean Goeurot, *The Regiment of lyfe* (London, 1567), sigs. A2v.

39 Phaire, "Preface to the Reader," sig. A2v.

40 Ann Rosalind Jones, *The Currency of Eros: Women's Love Lyric in Europe, 1540–1620* (Bloomington: Indiana University Press, 1990), 43–52; McGrath, *Subjectivity and Women's Poetry*, 152; Mary Ellen Lamb, "Isabella Whitney and the Travails of Service," (paper presented at the meeting of the Renaissance Society of America, Miami, Florida, March 24, 2007); Richard Panofsky, ed. The Floures of Philosophie *by Sir Hugh Plat*, vi–ix.

41 Wall, *The Imprint of Gender*, 310.

Clifford and Elizabeth Isham that held an herbal among various and more literary texts, I would like to suggest one more way of assessing Whitney's intertextuality; that is, Whitney shares language with texts that she has identified with hers *through analogy*. Whitney provides a metaphoric affordable "medicine" to her readership analogous to the actual remedies described in print herbal texts, and in thus framing her text, she shares an essential element found across print medical texts. From Lyte, Goeurot, and Moulton, we see authorial identification with the poor in the face of expensive physician care, and with this authorial stance we may gain insight into Whitney's choice of herbalism for her extended metaphor.

I may go so far as to contend that the poet's medical knowledge is an indicator that Whitney had an awareness of print medical materials, at least peripherally, because Whitney's vocabulary is not that of common parlance. Heretofore the emphasis on Whitney's medicine's roots in the domestic practice of women would seem to remove her knowledge from the public forum of print, but in presenting *Nosgay* in print in a vocabulary that comes from print, she invokes that very forum. Even though the poet does list several books she reads in the *Nosgay*, the author's library, as Wall has shown us, is not necessarily limited to those named books, and it is very possible that there are several more in the author's closet.[42] Plat's *Floures* may provide the inspiration for the volume and even the metaphor of the slips of flowers to present as a nosegay, but Whitney very likely consulted other texts in order to expand the medicinal metaphor in a concerted way. In particular, instances in which the poet addresses the variable humoral make-up (hot, cold, moist, dry) of individuals such as "as we are not all alyke, / nor of complexion one: / So that which helpeth some we see, / to others good doth none" (sig. A7r) and "if that thy complexion, with them doo not agree: / Refer them to some friend of thine, / tyll thou their vertue see" (sig. A7v), reflect a solid grounding in Galenic theory. Structural details in the poem also support this theory in that the poet's inclination to go for a walk and take air in the address to the reader also could come from Galen's medical treatments. She could have read the language of "complexion[s]" found throughout the address to the reader and come to understand the Galenic regimen that her persona undertakes in any number of medical texts from the period, but it is likely that she *read* it. That Galenic knowledge had to be learned and was not free-floating in the cultural atmosphere is evidenced by the many medical texts published throughout the sixteenth and seventeenth centuries, as surveyed at length by Paul Slack, Elizabeth Furdell, and Mary Fissell,[43] and it

---

42 For a discussion of Isabella Whitney's books, see Jones, *Currency of Eros*, 39.

43 Paul Slack, "Mirrors of Health and Treasures of Poor Men," 237–73; Elizabeth Lane Furdell, *Publishing and Medicine in Early Modern England* (Rochester, New York: University of Rochester Press, 2002); and Mary Fissell, *Patients, Power, and the Poor in Eighteenth-Century Bristol* (Cambridge: Cambridge University Press, 1991), and Fissell, "The Marketplace of Print," in *Medicine and the Market in England and Its Colonies*, ed. Mark S. R. Jenner and Patrick Wallis (Basingstoke, Hampshire: Palgrave Macmillan, 2007), 108–32. See also Harkness's depiction of the medical book trade in *The Jewel House*, 3.

is these texts that will provide a significant background for our understanding of Whitney's poetry.

Before looking at other medical texts, specifically those supplying herbal remedies, it is important to note that one critic before now has made a significant connection to texts providing medical advice and knowledge, yet only to a subset of the larger grouping. In an early analysis of Reniassance women writers, Kim Walker provides a possible textual precedent for Whitney's preventative medicine in Thomas Tusser's *A hundreth good pointes of Husbandry* (1570). In this intertextual connection, Walker offers a precursor for Whitney's physician Medicus, whose "counsel" the good housewife is to seek in creating medicines.[44] Importantly, Walker does not argue for Tusser as a source outright, but rather uses Tusser's wording to position Whitney's text, as others will do after her, within sixteenth-century constructions of "housewifery."[45] In thus highlighting this subgenre of texts supplying medical advice and with it Whitney's gender, Walker may exclude other potentials within the *Nosgay*, however. We have seen throughout this study how women who practiced medicine, whether within the household or beyond it, owned herbal texts other than those framed for women, and, in this chapter thus far, I hope I have demonstrated that the context of London and Whitney's persona as a poor woman without employment within that city problematizes any assumptions about the origins of Whitney's poetics within the household. In outlining the broader context of cheap print herbal texts, I intend to separate the poet's relationship to medical authority from questions of gender and allow for an alternate consideration of how this relationship is largely determined by economic and social status (only in part constituted by gender).

Through further surveying the herbal texts with which Whitney composes an analogous relationship, we will see more clearly how she positions herself relative to medical authority, particularly as it is varyingly embodied in cheap print medical texts and in the representations of the expensive physician found in them. Namely, I posit here that Whitney aligns her text not with the more costly folios read and treasured by English gentlewomen, but rather with the smaller texts meant to provide relief to a readership of lower economic status, a group of texts that have been studied at length by Furdell and Fissell, "popular," "cheap print," or "vernacular" medicine.[46] To uncover the specificities of the analogy Whitney develops, it will help us to consider further Whitney's relationship to her audience as it parallels-in-difference herbal texts of various sizes and costs.

---

44 Walker, *Women Writers*, 161.

45 See note 3, above.

46 Furdell, *Publishing and Medicine*; Mary Fissell, *Vernacular Bodies: The Politics of Reproduction in Early Modern England* (Oxford: Oxford University Press, 2004); Fissell, "The Marketplace of Print." See also Margaret Spufford, *Small Books and Pleasant Histories: Popular Fiction and Its Readership in Seventeenth-Century England* (Athens: The University of Georgia Press, 1981).

The analysis that follows reconsiders the context of print in an even more specific vein: Whitney's work not only appears in print, it does so in a small volume. As a work printed in octavo, Whitney's verses are likely to have been read by a wide-ranging readership. It follows that more affordable texts reached readers otherwise excluded by cost, but as Tessa Watt, as well as Fissell after her, has shown us, just because a work was more affordable does not mean that it played only to those of lesser financial means.[47] On the contrary, those works in the category of "cheap print"—pamphlets, broadsides, duodecimos, and octavos—reached the broadest audience possible. So while Whitney presents her text straightforwardly as a preventative for a plague-like disease of the mind, she also purveys a social critique for the amusement of—and perhaps against the behaviors of—some of her more elite readers, who are above her in status. Whitney may seem as if she presents a "simple gift" aimed at making her readership feel better, but her medicines prove to be much more complex.

We can see Whitney's specificity and complexity when we compare her use of "simple," as briefly discussed above, with that found in the "paratextual" elements, particularly in the addresses to the reader, of other herbal texts, as the paratexts most overtly articulate the relationship between author and reader.[48] The herbal texts to be examined are from all points in the spectrum of size and affordability, and by analyzing Whitney's use of this one word in this context, we can see how she establishes an analogous relationship not merely with herbal texts in general but with those of a particular size and with a particular audience construction. Whereas Whitney's use of "simple" sometimes serves as a pun and expresses a certain modesty in front of her readers of higher status, herbal texts of other purpose and higher cost use the word differently. They do so, however, always with an eye to their proposed readership, and it is through this similarity in difference that we can best understand Whitney's concerns.

Herbal Texts and the Simpler Audience

Given our extended acquaintance with them and their self-positioning as most authoritative, it makes sense to begin this brief survey with the folio herbals of Chapter 1. Long before John Parkinson changed the proposed title of his second volume from *The Garden of Simples* to *Theatrum Botanicum*, writers of folio herbals for the most part eschewed the term "simple" in their prefatory materials when referring to herbs in order to make their works seem more authoritative.[49]

---

[47] Tessa Watt, *Cheap Print and Popular Piety, 1550–1640* (Cambridge: Cambridge University Press, 1991); Fissell, *Vernacular Bodies*.

[48] Gérard Genette, *Paratexts: Thresholds of Interpretation*, trans. Jane E. Lewin (Cambridge: Cambridge University Press, 1997).

[49] Turner's use of "simple" in the letter to Elizabeth from *The first and seconde partes of the Herbal of William Turner Doctor in Phisick / lately ouersene / corrected and enlarged*

They did not, however, avoid the word when referring to uneducated (i.e., Latin-illiterate) herbal readers. The question of who was reading these hefty tomes is central to the prefatory materials in them, in that, on the one hand, the vernacular makes the books more readily accessible, while on the other, the authoritative weight (not to mention the expense) recognizes an elite readership. Nowhere is this bifurcated readership more apparent than in the 1562 dedicatory letter to Sir Thomas Wentworth from the second part of William Turner's herbal. In that dedication, Turner addresses detractors who "would haue only the mater simply told without any further examinacion and confutation of the errours that haue ben committed agaynst the knowledge of herbes / that I write of"[50] and in doing so, delineates a readership with two levels of education:

> I write not only this booke for vnlearned men / that as they care but littel for the truth / so can small skill of disputationes which are ordened for the defens of the truth / but also for lerned men / as surgeanes / apothecaries / and som Physiciones led away from the truth by the writinges of them / whom I go about to cōfute / had as much nede to haue the errours that they haue dronkē in / to be pulled out by disputationes / as the *simple* sorte haue nede only of the matter playnly told without any disputation at all. Therfore seying that both the *simple* writing of the matter is necessary / and the disputationes are necessary also / I am no more worthy blame for writing in one booke in som places *simply* the vertues and descriptiones of herbes / and in other places of the same disputationes and confutationes of errours / then the poore man is which bringeth an hole shepe to the market when as the clothier wold only by the wol / the glovers only the skin / and the inkeper the fleshe. (sigs. *2r–*2v, emphasis mine)

with the Third parte / lately gathered (Cologne, 1568) is a case in point. In a moment also quoted in Chapter 1, Turner juxtaposes his Elizabethan project with that of less advanced times, writing "suche was the ignorance in simples at that tyme / and as yet there was no Englishe herbal but one / al full of vnlearned cacographees and falselye naminge of herbes" (sig. *2v). The use of "simples" here would seem to be straightforward, meaning herbal medicines of one ingredient, except that its context causes one to wonder why Turner uses "simple" in such a way here and rarely in his other prefaces. In tying in the word "simples" with "the ignorance . . . at that tyme" and "unlearned cacographees," Turner seems to reflect that ignorance in the use of the word "simple." This reflection on the time (likely of *The Grete Herball* [1526]) of pre-Protestant England wants to signal the arrival of a true study of herbs, not "simply" a description of the uses of simples. Differently but nonetheless oxymoronically, John Gerard refers to the "rare simples" of Lord Burleigh's garden in his dedicatory letter; John Gerard, *The Herball or Generall Historie of Plantes* (London, 1597), sig. A2v.

50 William Turner, *The Seconde Part of VVilliam Turners Herball* (Cologne, 1562), sig. *2r. Virgules appear in the original text in lieu of punctuation. Subsequent references included in the text.

Turner's suggestion that the "simple sort" would not be interested in the disputations while "lerned men" might be most invested in such debates anticipates later projects, discussed below, that will excerpt the herbal virtues from the authoritative texts and leave behind the erudition. At the same time, this passage also acknowledges that the herbal has various uses and could not be limited to one readership. Turner's metaphor about the sheep at market seems to identify his detractors as those of the market, who would rather the book were smaller and thus more affordable. The physician-herbalist's response to them is that he intends his readership to be of multiple economic strata and educational levels, thus widest and most diverse. Of course, the contradiction of Turner's argument is that perhaps poorer men, as a result, would not be able to buy the folio volume because of higher costs resulting from its comprehensiveness. Regardless, Turner himself seems most invested in maintaining the interest of his learned English and continental counterparts.

As we have seen in Chapter 1, the folio herbals of Turner, Rembert Dodoens (as translated by Henry Lyte), John Gerard, and John Parkinson reveal the tensions that exist in the establishment of the English tradition. In their purported authoritative and comprehensive nature, these texts spoke to a professional audience that stood to gain from a more complete herbal knowledge. Appearing in print and written in English, however, these texts addressed wider concerns of accessibility. Through the comprehensive and authoritative vernacular herbal, knowledge once confined to the university-educated now belonged to every English-literate person. With this new accessibility came layers of readership that had to be accommodated, or at least accounted for. Introducing the only authoritative vernacular herbals printed before Whitney's *Nosgay*, Turner's front matter reveals that the size and thus the cost of the text may be prohibitive for a poorer readership.

A slightly later folio provides a different perspective on the question, however. Unlike Turner, Henry Lyte is not presenting in *A Nievve Herball* the results of his own original work but rather a translation of Dodoens, and as a result, his letter "To the friendly and indifferent Reader" quoted above has a different tenor (perhaps freer from authorial anxiety); however, it is no less reflective on the implications of herbal publication. Like Turner's, Lyte's preface anticipates his critics, but in Lyte's imaginings, the critics want to make access to herbal knowledge less available. Lyte's response, syntactically tangled as it may be, is one that regards the greed of certain physicians who want to make the general populace subject to their expertise:

> Seing then y^t my translation shall make this good & profitable historie (whiche hitherto hath lien hid from many of my Countriemen, vnder the vayle of an vnknowen language) familiar and knowen vnto them: and if it be good …to enlarge a good thing, and to make many partakers thereof: then can there not lacke iust cause to be alleaged of this my doyng: neither thinke I, that any will mislike or repine therat, except such, as either envie the Weale of others whom they accompt *simpler* then them selues, and therfore recken vnworthy to be in their owne language made partakers therof: or els are so studious of their owne

> priuate gaine, that they feare, least by this meanes some parte therof may be lessened: whyles others vnderstanding the nature and vertues of Plantes and herbes, shalbe the lesse beholding to their scrupulous skill.[51]

Lyte turns from the image of the greedy physician preying on the uneducated and desperate that recurs in sixteenth-century English culture to the quote from earlier in this discussion, the parenthesis of which describes "the meanest of [his] Countriemen," "whose skill is not so profounde that they can fetche . . . knowledge out of strange tongues, nor their habilities so wealthy, as to entertaine a learned Phisition."[52] The author outlines the economics of his endeavor: again, stated simply, while the folio herbal may have been relatively costly for a book, it is a minor expense when it comes to the fee of "a learned Phisition." The author's use of "simpler" suggests a hierarchy of readership implicit throughout these works and shows how despite this hierarchy, when presented in the vernacular, herbal knowledge is available to a much wider audience and, by extension, leads to broader lay practice.

Historians of medicine have noted the equalizing aspects in the mid-seventeenth-century works of Nicholas Culpeper's volumes, citing the influence of the Levelers' arguments about equal access to the law on Culpeper's medical publications.[53] In terms of the religious correlation, they also discuss the parallels Culpeper makes between the English translation of the pharmaceutical recipes of the College of Physicians and that of the Bible, quoting the contention in the preface to *Culpeper's School of Physick* (1659) that "there are not such slaves to the Doctors, as the poor English are; most of them profess themselves Protestants, but their practices have been like those of the Papists, to hide the grounds of Physick from the vulgar."[54] Indeed, as Andrew Wear, Mary Fissell, and Elizabeth Furdell have shown, this "leveling" spirit preceded the civil war in examples such as Thomas Elyot, Stephen Bradwell, and Henry Lyte, and many medical texts cite equal economic access (aside from economic gain) as their prime motivator.[55] Both Fissell and Furdell have discussed the ethos of "Every Man His Own Doctor" that surrounded these volumes, and even the most expensive of these expressed the economic implications of such an enterprise. Correspondingly, as books became more affordable, the equalizing potentials of these publications gained a prominent position within the prefatory materials.[56]

---

51 Henry Lyte, "To the friendly and indifferent Reader," sig. *3r, emphasis mine.

52 Lyte, "To the friendly and indifferent Reader," sig. *3r.

53 Fissell, *Vernacular Bodies*, 137–41; Hill, "The Medical Profession and Its Radical Critics"; Andrew Wear, *Knowledge and Practice in English Medicine, 1550–1680* (Cambridge: Cambridge University Press, 2000).

54 As quoted in Wear, *Knowledge and Practice*, 44, n. 84.

55 Wear, *Knowledge and Practice*; Fissell, *Patients, Power and the Poor*; Furdell, *Publishing and Medicine.*

56 Fissell, *Patients, Power, and the Poor*; Furdell, *Publishing and Medicine*, 49–74.

While Turner and Lyte addressed critics from different levels of readership, in essence the assumptions they had were very similar; that is, given the authority of their work—Turner's in his own experiments and erudition and Lyte's in his Continental source—physicians, apothecaries, and surgeons would be reading and consulting their volumes. As creators of authoritative texts, however, their engagement with the vernacular—both projects being framed in proto-nationalistic terms as explored in Chapter 1—invited another level of readership. In their prefatory materials, these herbalists recognized and even defended this readership that existed outside the "tripartite division of medicine" and included women.[57] So while they targeted England's physicians, apothecaries, and surgeons as the primary audience for their volumes, they had to accommodate the necessary presence of readers existing outside this three-part medical structure who saw the herbal as a tool for more affordable healthcare. It is the language of "simple" that registers tensions around the economic and educational disparity of medical care in sixteenth-century England.

Central to any discussion of these disparities has been the ongoing historical debate about the literacy rate of the "simple sort" and the difficulties of its determination. While this debate—in which measurable pieces of evidence such as signatures in loyalty oaths prove unsatisfactory and other kinds of evidence somewhat anecdotal[58]—directly informs our discussion in this chapter, we may now consider that the subject of the "simpler" reader and the subject of different levels of literacy have been with us all along. In Chapter 1, we have seen how Turner dismisses the possibility that the "old wife," because illiterate, could use his herbal for profit, marking her illiteracy as a sign of the unreliability of her knowledge. Then in Chapter 2, Ann Parsons acquires writing literacy at the same time as she encounters the herbal, and in the chapter previous to this one, Elizabeth Isham eschews "learned" status in acquiring Latin for a solid medical knowledge base derived largely from the authoritative vernacular herbals. As I could not through these previous examples, I will not attempt here to resolve any ongoing determinations but rather merely want to point out that in our consideration of smaller print medical texts, we see that the paratextual elements in them target an audience of the poor and unlearned, thus giving evidence to a non-elite—if unnamed and unknowable—readership. When Isabella Whitney, furthermore,

---

[57] Margaret Pelling, "Trade or Profession? Medical Practice in Early Modern England," *The Common Lot: Sickness, Medical Occupations and the Urban Poor in Early Modern England* (Harlow, Essex: Longman, 1998), 235. See my discussion of the vulnerability and instability of this construction in the introduction above.

[58] David Cressy's analysis of signature statistics stands at the center of renditions and extensions of the debate; David Cressy, *Literacy and the Social Order: Reading and Writing in Tudor and Stuart England* (Cambridge: Cambridge University Press, 1980). For a long summary of and thoughtful engagement with the literacy debate, see Heidi Brayman Hackel, *Reading Material in Early Modern England: Print, Gender, and Literacy* (Cambridge: Cambridge University Press, 2005), 55–68.

identifies herself as "simple" and signifies her reading of small medical texts, she places herself in the category of the uncounted and thus gives us insight into the non-elite readership position. Again, in this study's emphasis on the individual reader, we can differentiate between various readers through their contexts.

These "small books" consistently carve out an audience position—poor individual in need of medicine—that the poet comes to occupy in her persona and then to recreate in her reader construction. Thus in the examples of Turner and Lyte, we see a different use of the word "simple" than we have in Whitney's *Nosgay*. Neither Turner nor Lyte use the word in deference to a patron or more elite readership, nor do they present their folio works as a "simple gift" to someone above them in the social strata. As Protestant physician and well-established herbalist respectively, each of these men anticipates an audience of peers, and their authoritative works are too large to be labeled "simple." Whitney's use of the word reveals an author who presents a small work to a large populace, many of whom are above her in status. Her use of "simple" thus denotes a hierarchy in which the author exists close to the bottom rather than a hierarchy conceived by the writer from the privileged vantage of "author." This difference is crucial in understanding the nature of Whitney's critique and her cure.

Before turning to smaller books closer to Whitney's, let us consider another text occupying an intermediary position that illuminates other aspects of an herbal's relationship to authority. Existing in quarto and from two decades later, William Langham's *Garden of health* (1597/8), derived largely from the authoritative herbals, employs the language of "simple" to very different effect.[59] Without the disputations and etymologies seen in Turner, Dodoens, and Gerard, the purpose of Langham's volume is clear: to provide an easily negotiated and relatively affordable herbal for practical use. Reflecting this straightforward purpose is the plain use of "simple" in his letter to the reader:

> In this booke are conteined very many & strange effects and operations of all sorts of *simples*, gathered by the long experience and trauaile of the Authour, so that for variety of things therein handled, it may be compared with any that are written of the like argument. All which *simples* with their vses are easily knowen, being plainely described in this booke, and are gotten without any great cost or labour, the most of them being such as growe in most places, and are common amongst vs. But for thy better direction, thou shalt vnderstand (good Reader) that all the *simples* . . . are set downe in order of the Alphabet, so that thou mayest without any difficulty finde them by the titles of the pages: and to euery *simple* is annexed a briefe Tabel of effects thereof. There are moreouer

[59] William Langham, *The Garden of health, Conteyning the sundry rare and hidden vertues and properties of all kindes of Simples and Plants* (London, 1597/8). Several examples of this volume I have seen have changed the 1597 date to 1598, indicating that it was published in the early months of our modern calendar's 1598. This date follows from its gleanings from Gerard's larger volume.

> two generall Tables: the one at the beginning of the booke, conteining all the *simples* in order, with numbers directing to the seuerall places where they are to bee found: the other at the ende setting downe the names of the diseases and other operations, hauing those *simples* which afford any remedy for the same, added vnto them in order so plainely, as thou canst not erre therein.[60]

In this brief epistle, Langham uses the word "simple" six times, every time meaning the same thing, a single herb of medicinal use. Also noteworthy is Langham's use of synonyms for "simple" in its other meanings: "plaine[ly]," "without any great cost or labour," "easily knowen," "common amongst us," and "without any difficulty." In essence, this book of simples is simple, and Langham seems to go out of his way to avoid the pun that would complicate his relationship to his project and his readership. That is, when it is used by others to emphasize its economic and educational associations, the word "simple" implies a social order and requires an educated and rich foil to impart its judgment. Importantly, all of the instances before this one designate a hierarchy: between Turner's "unlearned" and "lerned" men, between the physician and "the meanest of . . . Countriemen," and between Isabella Whitney and her brother, married sister, former employer, and patron. Langham's plain use of "simple" implies a non-hierarchized readership and shows an equality of address. Sold directly to his reader for clear and easy access to knowledge, his herbal seems to have no patron. While not the least expensive herbal available, Langham's is a work with one application and purpose—to be used in practice. Purged of *disputatio*, it is less expensive than the folios from which it is derived.

In some ways, volumes such as Langham's return the herbal to its pre-Turner format found in *The Grete Herbal* (1516/26) and Anthony Askham's *Lytel herball* (1550), volumes that are derivative of their precursors and intent on simply spreading herbal knowledge, but the effect of the intercession of the English herbal tradition as established by Turner and his followers and the consequent drive for a comprehensive and authoritative herbal in English is that such derivation is now less about vernacular access and more about economic access.[61] The most overt testimony to this beyond Langham's preface is the existence of *Rams Little Dodeons* [*sic*], *a brief epitome of the new herbal or history of plantss* (1606), authored by a William Ram, which has barely any relation to Lyte's translation but nonetheless markets itself through its comparative littleness (and affordability).[62] With these derivative volumes in mind, we may gain further insight into Whitney's volume. Whitney presents her collection as derivative of Hugh Plat's larger quarto, so in part it is analogous to a work such as Langham's in that hers is a smaller

---

60 Langham, *The Garden of health*, sigs. A2r–A2v.

61 Eleanour Sinclair Rohde gives a clarifying account of English herbal history in *The Old English Herbals* (1922, reprint New York: Dover Publications, Inc., 1971).

62 William Ram, *Rams Little Dodeons* [sic], *a brief epitome of the new herbal or history of plants* (London, 1606).

volume that holds similar and selected "flowers." Alternatively, her work may have more in common with *Rams Little Dodeons* as very little is in actuality Plat's; she expands and adds her own poems, many of which give advice.

At some level, all small herbals are selected and derivative—the purpose of the folios' bulk being their motivation for comprehensiveness—and it is through this selectivity, as we have in part seen in the Bulckley volume discussed in the introduction, that they gain specificity and personality. Thus the mistake would be to assume that the smaller the herbal, the more bare-bones it becomes. Even though Langham's quarto text has less authorial presence than the folios, smaller texts are not necessarily less encumbered by authorial mediation. Evidence to this point is the smallest of the print herbals, Philip Moore's duodecimo *The hope of Health wherein is conteined a goodlie regimente of life: as medecine, good diet, and the goodlie vertues of Sonderie herbes* (1565), which contains an author's address "to the gentill Reader" and a dedicatory epistle to "the right VVorshipfull Sir Owen Hopton knight." Indeed Moore's textual persona has much in common with Whitney's; in his address to the reader and his dedicatory epistle, Moore puns on "simple" in a manner similar to Whitney's, referring to the "simple labours of mine" (labors in simples) in the former and, again, "this simple gifte" and "my simple trauaile" in the latter.[63] This coincidence occurs because, in his text, unlike those of Lyte and Langham, Moore positions himself below his "gentle reader" and his patron. Thus it is in "cheap print" medical texts that we see similar hierarchies of readership to what we have witnessed in Whitney's *Nosgay*.

We can best expand on the economic implications of these hierarchies through an octavo text containing much knowledge about herbs, William Bullein's *A newe booke Entituled the Gouernement of Health wherein is vttred manye notable Rules for mannes preseruacion, with sondry symples & other matters, no lesse fruiteful then profitable: colect out of many approued authours. Reduced into the forme of Dialogue, for the better vnderstanding of thunlearned*, first published in 1558/9. After the title page, Bullein presents the dedicatory epistle to his patron Sir Thomas Hilton, and after his initial address "To the gentle Reader," he turns to the "gentle reader" again after the final page in presenting a list of errata.[64] The gentry are not Bullein's only audience, however, and evidence of this fact exists in the full title, "the unlearned," for whom the dialogue structure is conceived. The two main characters, John and Humfrey, are a young and foolish pursuer of pleasures and an older and wise physician, respectively. More reminiscent of many religious catechisms of the period than humanist colloquies, Bullein's text presents the

---

[63] Philip Moore, *The hope of Health wherein is conteined a goodlie regimente of life: as medecine, good diet, and the goodlie vertues of Sonderie herbes* (London, 1565), n.p.

[64] William Bullein, *A newe boke Entituled the Gouernement of Health: wherein is vttred manye notable Rules for mannes preseruacion, with sondry symples and other matters, no lesse fruitfull then profitable* (London, 1559).

material in dialogue for better understandability.[65] We can also read this format as diffusing the presence of the author and audience within the personas presented. Bullein, himself a physician in Durham and Northumberland,[66] creates his persona "Humfrey the wise" (n.p.), a figure for the good physician and a kindly counselor, through whom the author, as physician, can instill his advice. So the volume thus presents three levels of readership above, equal to, and beneath the author in status in the figure of Sir Thomas, in the discernment of the "gentle" reader, and in John, the reader in need of the physician's counsel.

Gouernement, like *Hope of Health*, has much in common with *Sweet Nosgay* in its use of "simple." In the poetic envoy to Lord Hilton, we see that the author uses the word unmistakably as a person of lesser means bowing to his benefactor, and in doing so, he puts his benefactor in line with his medical predecessors, Hippocrates, Galen, Dioscorides, Avicenna (Persian physician), and Pliny, the "them" of the first line:

> To them I bend my knee with dewe reuerence,
> As one unworthy their fotesteppes for to kisse,
> Lacking no good will confessing my negligence,
> Though many will iudge, my entent amisse.
> Powring water in the sea, where aye plentie is.
> But of your worship to whome I present this gift,
> Except it better thē nothing to make a *simple* shift.
> (sig. A6v, emphasis mine)

Then, in prose, Bullein presents his book to the "gentle reader" in a way that should remind us of the way Whitney gives her nosegay to her audience, framed as an act of good will for the "happy healthe of mankynde." Bullein writes, "Here I doe present vnto thee (gentle Reader) a symple Gouernemēt of helth, beseching thee moste heartely for to except it as an argument of my good wyll, as one unfaynedly that greatly dooe couit the good fate and happy healthe of mankynde" (sig. A7r). We could read the resonances with Whitney here and in Moore's text as coincidental playing upon the same pun, but even this coincidence carries meaning within a given context. While the folios address issues of a "simpler" readership accessing learned materials and Langham's text avoids the pun, Whitney, Moore, and Bullein couch their projects in modesty while presenting their texts as "simple" medicine for the benefit of the collective readership's health. The hierarchies of readership function differently within the folios than in the smaller texts, and the

---

65 For comparison, see William Roye, "The Catechism in Sixteenth-Century England," introductory material to *A Brefe Dialoge Bitwene a Christen Father and his Stobborne Sonne: The First Protestant Catechism Published in English* (Toronto: University of Toronto Press, 1999), 23–49.

66 Patrick Wallis, "Bullein, William (c. 1515–1576)," *DNB*, http://www.oxforddnb.com/view/article/3910 (accessed September 11, 2006).

use of "simple" in each points to that dissimilarity. Even though the stance of modesty and the administration of herbal remedy mean differently across gender lines, the coincidence of the language of "simple" in these smaller texts shows that there is a precedent for Whitney's topos that is neither gendered female nor located in the domestic.

Instead, my argument again posits that Whitney's herbalism, beyond placing her in the context of charitable and domestic work, positions her within the larger realm of social critique found throughout cheap print medical texts. These critiques castigate physicians for their high costs while warning their readers about the neglect of their health. In her very poverty, Whitney's persona aligns herself with a discussion that is neither authoritative nor established but rather one that is necessary and critical. Her work, while infused with "good will," also disapproves of certain social truths. So while she may articulate a fear of censure by the power structures, she finds a way of being critical of those structures, making this more than a simple narrative of subjugation as well. The nature of Whitney's criticism as of yet may remain unclear, and these subtleties in her verse can be further illuminated through one more small medical text, one that provides a satire of the London context at the same time as it proffers various herbal preventatives against the plague.

Whitney's Herbal Satire

Between the first publication of Bullein's *Gouernement* and that of *Nosgay*, one quarter of London's population, most of whom were poor, died in the summer of 1563. While London and its deadly summer cannot figure in Moore's *Hope of Health* or Bullein's *Gouernement* (both of which are comparatively optimistic), they do prominently in Whitney's text and in a later book by Bullein, *A Dialogve bothe pleasaunte and pietifull, wherein is a goodly regimente against the feuer Pestilence with a consolacion and comfort against death* (1564). Bullein wrote *A Dialogve* a year after the plague, when he had moved closer to London and after he had been put through the societal wringer in a scandal surrounding Sir Thomas Hilton's death and Bullein's marriage with his widow. Bullein composed his popular *Dialogve*[67]—published again in 1573 and 1578—in Edward Barrett's

[67] An early twentieth-century editor of the *Dialogve* writes that "being full of merry tales (pills to purge the melancholy at plague-time), [it] is one of those books that are most easily thumbed out of existence" and quotes Thomas Nashe's invocation of the text in *Haue with you to Saffron Walden* as evidence of its popularity as late as 1596, Mark W. Bullen and A. H. Bullen, eds., "Note," *A Dialogue against the Feuer Pestilence / by William Bullein; from the Edition of 1578, Collated with Earlier Editions of 1564 and 1573*, n.p.. Edition referred to here, William Bullein, *A Dialogve bothe pleasaunte and pietifull, wherein is a goodly regimente against the feuer pestilence with a consolacion and comfort against death* (London, 1564).

home in Essex, adjacent to the plague-wary city of London. Indeed, dedicating the book to Barrett, he sets the *Dialogve* in London proper; though it is not named, a character's reference to "a reformed and godly city named 'Nodnol,'" implies that the opposite of the "reformed and godly" is that city's name backwards.[68] The first character we meet, Mendicus, is a beggar displaced from Northumberland (Bullein's former home) by enclosure. The references to the conditions "in the citee" (fol. 4r) are colored by images of children being carried out into the countryside to escape the plague and of unwholesome physicians who charge exorbitant fees for ineffectual medicine to those who remain in the city. By contrast with his earlier sage Humfrey, Bullein presents healers who are much less reputable. The characters we meet have spent lifetimes steeped in greed and avarice. This is early modern London.

Whereas Bullein's *Gouernement of Health* overtly addressed only a "gentle readership" as it censured a nondescript epicure through a wise physician, the *Dialogve* includes elements that seem to appeal more openly to readers of lower status. The author's general address is to the "Good" rather than the "Gentle" reader, and the content of the volume is much more satirical of the wealthy than Bullein's earlier octavo work. Whereas the generic epicure John in *Gouernement* converts to Humfrey's point of view very quickly and easily with Humfrey's account of a plague death, much of the *Dialogve*—in fulfillment of its preface, exposes "the mercilesse rich, whose whole trust is in the vaine riches of this world, entangled as it were emong Briers" (sig. A2v), and shows the parasitic system of law and medicine that surrounds them. The poverty of Mendicus, the greed of Antonius (the sick merchant at the center of the text), and the corruption of the physician and apothecary attending him all point to a very different worldview than *Gouernement*.

When considering the satirical edge of this work, one may be surprised to find correspondences with Whitney's sweet and wholesome *Nosgay*, but certain shared elements show us that Whitney's work, published in the same year *Dialogve* was first republished, goes beyond the good will found in *Gouernement*. I want to argue that it may be Bullein's later text that provided the model for preventative regimen because it is in this text that we also find the element of social critique. Within the frame of the satirical dialogue, Bullein provides a literal precedent for Whitney's metaphoric preventative medicine in several pages of herbal recipes to stave off the plague, including a perfume and a pomander, and others to alleviate its symptoms (fols. 35v–38v). Though none are made simply of flowers, those of "sweete" scent include roses, lilies, and violets (fol. 37r) and other plant-based ingredients. For its social critique, Whitney's *Nosgay* may also find a model in Bullein's *Dialogve* more than any of the other print medical texts from the period. Very early in Whitney criticism, Elaine Beilin identified the "satirical look" in Whitney's "Wyll and Testament" at "the conspicuous consumption of the lords,

68 Wallis, "Bullein," 2.

ladies, and gentlefolk,"[69] and I assert here that it is through a possible allusion to Bullein's *Dialogve* that we can see that this satire begins in *Nosgay* as early as the address to her reader.

Lightly in *Gouernement* and fully in *Dialogve*, Bullein censures the rich, who, in the pursuit of wealth, do not "regard their health"—both physical and spiritual—until it is too late, when they have been infected and are brought to death's door. We find this critique in *Gouernement* only in the addresses to Sir Thomas, through their allusions to the Bible and to Diogenes. As much of the *Dialogve* centers upon this critique of the wealthy, however, the years of social strife and the move closer to plague-ridden London seem to have infected Bullein's outlook; his merchant Antonius, who has spent his life in pursuit of earthly riches, contracts the plague, becomes aware of his own imminent damnation, and seeks desperately for a cure. His physician, known in the *dramatis personae* and throughout the dialogue as "Medicus" (distinct from his beggar Mendicus, the representative poor person, who does not share the stage with the doctor), gives him spiritual counsel but not before he leeches fees from his patient for useless drugs, enemas, and bloodlettings, aligning him with the greedy physician and the "merchant" doctor from Lyte's and Phaire's prefaces. In the course of the dialogue, we find that Medicus is related to the allegorical lawyer Avarus, who hovers around the rich man's deathbed like a Jonsonian vulture, and after Medicus's apothecary, Crispinus, has moral qualms and vows to "caste awaie a greate nomber of rotten drugges" (fol. 20r) that he was selling as viable, Medicus whispers to him, "The vicar of sainct fooles bee your ghostlie father . . . tary still with me, let hym paie for your rotten drugges, for I maie saie to you, that he is almost rotten alreadie hymself" (fol. 20r–20v). Again, this popular image of the physician in London is reprinted in 1573.

And it is with this physician that we find the most overt, and arguably conclusive, connection to Whitney's poet, who tells her reader, "yf thy mind infected be, / then these wyll not prevayle / Sir *Medicus* with stronger Earbes, / thy malladye must quayle" (sigs. A7r–A7v), and continues, "For these be but to keepe thee sound, / which if thou use them well: / (Paynes of my lyfe) in healthy state / thy mind shall ever dwell" (sig. A7v). This language of prevention pervades the *Nosgay* volume: in her address to the reader (as she herself is advised to leave the dirty streets of London and as she provides the nosegay as preventative medicine), in flowers 18 ("For libertye doth lewdnesse breed, / wherfore prevent that yll" [sig. B3v]) and 96 ("He doth not soone to ruyne come / that feares it ere it fall" [sig. C3v]), in her prescriptive letter to her younger sisters, and in the final description of Londoners who "bathe themselves, so to prevent / infection of the ayre" (sig. E5r). Although this language has been in part analyzed by Kim Walker in her discussion of Thomas Tusser's handbook and the woman's role in the first line of medical care,[70] my analysis differs from Walker's in showing that Whitney's emphasis on

[69] Beilin, *Redeeming Eve*, 99. See also Ellinghausen, "Literary Property and the Single Woman," 14.

[70] Walker, *Women Writers*, 161.

prevention reflects the language of health regimens in general and not just those prescribed for women's practice. In a text such as Bullein's the message is clear: the best way to cure the plague is not to get it in the first place. Whitney's directive to her reader who is already infected could then be an admonition: you have not fortified yourself, so your only recourse is a futile one, Sir Medicus's "stronger Earbes," which for those who know their Bullein means "rotten drugges." While admittedly this connection between Medicus figures is not entirely incontrovertible, it is important that readers of Whitney consider the context of *Dialogve* and like-minded texts because of the potentials that they introduce. Specifically, the figure of Bullein's Medicus presents an alternative to the domestic reading proposed by Walker and the housewife's deference to good Medicus in Tusser's household manual. The existence of an alternative opens up the text to multivalency rather than restricting Whitney and her persona to the housewife's role. In the cohabitation with Bullein's text, Whitney's Medicus seems a less-than-exemplary figure and *Nosgay* seems less deferential toward licensed medical authority. In this reading, the "Sir" would not be a courtesy but a slur and an indication of his high cost and the status of his clientele.

Indeed, the critique of the rich and the identification with the poor can be found throughout Whitney's text (and her chosen source in Plat), in flowers such as number 60, "The poore, they have no frends at al / for to participate, / The sorow and the griefe they finde / in their most wretched state" (sig. B8r), and, as articulated by Beilin, is seen most overtly in the "Wyll and Testament," in which Whitney's persona is one without employment and who is "very weake in Purse" (sig. E3r). Even though the poet cannot access the rich "banquets" that London has to offer, she shows us that this superfluous feasting leads many of these consumers, whom she describes as "daynty mouthes . . . and stomacks weake," to the apothecary's shop and the physician's door (sig. E4v). The word "dainty," as we have seen in Chapter 1, carries with it all of the connotations of wealth and vanity that imbue the rest of the passage. In leaving London, she stands outside its excesses.

Thus "Sir Medicus" is a figure that belongs to London. The city readers, who frequent the same booksellers as Whitney represents in the "Wyll," would recognize him as a figure both above and beneath them and as someone who carries the knowledge to heal but who is also corrupted by that knowledge. The London the poet leaves at the end of the volume is one riddled with disease, poverty, and avaricious mercantilism. It is the same London as found in Bullein's *Dialogve*.

In this juxtaposition of Whitney's nosegay to Sir Medicus's herbs, of her collection of healthful flowers to his "rotten drugges," the poet's herbal frame provides a means of engaging concerns about high costs and consequent corruption in London, while giving a means of support to those who are downtrodden by the system. In not naming her herbs, Whitney does not make her herbalism more abstract but rather allows for the possibilities behind the signifiers that go beyond gender and beyond "kitchen physic." Her poetic herbs do not simply reference a generic women's practice that stands respectfully in front of licensed medical authority, but rather challenge the motivations and efficacy of that authority when and where it is most needed. As a result, her poetry draws on literal concerns about equal access to healthcare and the corrupt sources of that care in order to expand her metaphoric critique. The high cost of healthcare is but one concern for a poor woman unemployed and vulnerable in London. Ultimately, the preventative medicine she offers considers the disease surrounding the sickness, and in leaving the center of that disease and sickness at the end of the volume, she offers a most effective preventative medicine to her readership in bitter satirical terms. In this way, the entirety of the 1573 text serves as a metaphoric herbal nosegay for her reader in the protection it offers through the critical eye it has on London's economy and the model it provides in the poet's leaving it behind.

In engaging more affordable herbal texts, Whitney's use of herbalism signifies differently from that of Hoby, Mildmay, and Isham. As a result, her articulated relationship to the licensed physician differs from theirs as well, even as Hoby, Mildmay, and Isham vary from each other. In essence, no two of these women reference herbalism in the same way or construct the same relationship to licensed authority. In articulating their geographic, marital, and economic positions, these women have provided many lenses through which to view their herbs, and through similar lenses and others not here described, we may further appreciate other examples that come to our attention. The simple statement of the fact that women practiced medicine in early modern England is not adequate to understanding the nuances of each text, and I hope that this study has presented a model for pursuing the intricacies of herbal—and perhaps other—language.

In developing my focus here on women's direct engagement with herbal medical texts, I have had to exclude other examples, some more obvious (i.e., Ann Wheathill's prayerbook *A handfull of holesome (though homelie) hearbs*) than others, from my consideration. That the examples in this study all engage at some level herbal texts through their herbal language is what brings them together. We may find in further research that sometimes an herbal reference may point to a group of texts that are not primarily medical in their nature but are rather devotional (which is the case with Wheathill), philosophical, or poetical, or (as with Whitney's use of both Plat and Bullein) such a reference may point to two or more texts that, however generically different, overlap in their use of herbal language. Then again, in many instances other texts may not be involved and the text may reflect a more direct engagement with the plants themselves. Regardless, we should not think it enough to gloss any example as merely reflective of a general gendered material reality. Rather, each herbal reference should be taken on its own terms. Often these terms are intertextual, sometimes not; importantly, we should not fixate on a cultural practice that would not create a stir in the early modern breast, as scintillating as we may find it. Yes, women practiced medicine in early modern England, but how much more interesting that they wrote about it, bought books in support of it, and even transformed it to meet their own rhetorical ends.

In conducting our rhetorical analysis of such instances, the strongest determining textual factor in discerning meaning in women's herbalism has been the generic differences in the works studied. Even within the one category of autobiographical writings, as we have seen with the help of Sharon Seelig's study, there are different ways of reading and representing authoritative herbals, and in considering Whitney's poetic satire, we have witnessed again how the constellation of herbal texts creates potential for cultural critique and multiple tonal meanings through the motif of herbalism. Exploring yet other genres may help extend my analysis beyond these pages, as genre may indicate potentials in allusion and direct intertextual engagement that complicate and expand women's textual applications of herbalism.

In any case, a close analysis of early modern women's engagements with herbal texts through their writing will go beyond what is "inscribed in the text" for the general female practitioner, as the contours of each life, whether historical or fictional, are as expandable and changeable as the social networks to which that life belongs.[71] So another aspect of the writings by Hoby, Mildmay, Isham, and Whitney that ultimately distinguishes them from others is the fact that each text supplies an autobiographical construct, which then provides the context for developing understanding. As we have seen in examples such as Compiler A from the Bulckley text, however, such overt life contexts are not always readily available. With regard to such instances, I hope that we have begun to see how most every moment presents some difference that may further our understanding of the perspective involved. That is, every reference to women's herbs comes with a context, and articulating that context allows us to discern the particularities of the herbal language concerned.

In the final analysis, one hope I have for this work is that its articulation of another kind of network may be extended through further study—and not only my own continued research with women's medical texts. As I found the examples of women's herbal ownership scattered throughout the United States and Great Britain, it became clear to me that my book could serve as a kind of "call-out," asking for future scholars to keep Appendix B with them as they perform their own digs through the archives. Provenance records are a rarity still, and even when these records exist, each must be brought into dialogue with others. As I conducted my research, I began to imagine what it would mean for Mistress X's herbal to find her recipe book, her Paracelsian treatise, or—a grail-like imagining—her autobiography. I began to see how different scholars in pursuit of their own fragments would come upon the puzzle pieces that interested others. I am thankful for the conversations that have realized these potentials through their generosity,[72] and for the innumerable librarians whose loving consideration of their collections have connected me with those of others.

---

71 Chartier, *Cultural History*, 13.

72 I am thankful particularly for conversations, both virtual and in person, with Karen Reeds and Elaine Leong, who have been looking at herbals and other print medical texts for different ends alongside me.

As women's libraries continue to surface through newly discovered signatures, inventories, wills, and life-writings, patterns may emerge that could well be worth pursuing. Herbals constitute but one kind of text that repeatedly appears in early modern women's closets, and we may find that each kind of text, even each specific text, can open up another array of textual and intertextual potentials. Early modern libraries may also point us to variation within a certain kind of text, as the more authoritative and expensive resides next to the smaller and more concise. This kind of relative valuing and the kinds of social variables that may come with it—be they doctrinal, political, economic, or aesthetic—lead to numerous modes of differentiation. As we consider women's representation of other kinds of specialized knowledge—such as gardening, alchemy, preserve making, needlework, biblical exegesis, and poetry writing (all of which have come in contact with our discussion of herbalism)—we no longer limit women's writings (and the objects that may accompany them) within a small space of knowing.[73] In the details of each frame of reference, we encounter again the infinite variety within the workings of creative minds.

[73] I have been referring to works on these and related fields throughout this study. For examples, see Jennifer Munroe, *Gender and the Garden in Early Modern English Literature* (Burlington, Vermont: Ashgate Publishing, 2008); Susan Frye, "Sewing Connections: Elizabeth Tudor, Mary Stuart, Elizabeth Talbot, and Seventeenth-Century Anonymous Needleworkers," in *Maids and Mistresses, Cousins and Queens: Women Alliances in Early Modern England*, ed. Susan Frye and Karen Robertson (New York: Oxford University Press, 1999), 165–182; Jane Stevenson, *Women Latin Poets: Language, Gender, and Authority, from Antiquity to the Eighteenth Century* (Oxford: Oxford University Press, 2005). The ongoing but yet unpublished work of Kate Narveson on Mildmay's readings of scripture also provides inspiration in its analogy.

Appendix A
Translating Artemisia

Even decisions of translation and appropriation made by the four herbal authors are informed by gender politics. The herbal entries themselves, specifically with regard to the herb artemisia (also known as "mugwort"), show how classical precedent may be manipulated over time and within certain situations.

The prefatory materials of both Lyte and Gerard draw our attention to the herb artemisia. In duplication of Dodoens' 1554 Flemish edition (a context discussed below), Lyte's frontispiece represents Queen Artemisia of Caria, associated with the herb of that name.[1] In the top right corner of a royal square, she is an interesting figure (see Figure 2.1). Unlike her male counterparts—labeled "Gentius" (top left), "Methridates" (bottom left), and "Lysimachus" (bottom right)—who are also rulers who have contributed to herbal knowledge, she faces outward and looks despondent, holding an unidentifiable flower. This image refers to two parts of her legend: the flower refers to her position in the herbal tradition; her despondency is something else altogether. The source of her sorrow can be found in such accounts as that of Christine de Pizan:

> Of all the ladies who have loved their husbands devotedly and who have demonstrated their love in fact, I would like to add, regarding that noble lady Artemisia, queen of Caria, that, just as was said above, insofar as she had followed King Mausolus into so many battles and was stricken and overcome with as much grief as anyone could bear when he died, she showed no less devotion in the end than she had demonstrated during his lifetime. . . . [D]uring a dignified funeral in the presence of the princes and barons, she had his body cremated. She herself gathered his ashes together, washing them with her tears before she placed them in a gold vessel. Now it struck her that there was no reason why the ashes of the man whom she had so loved should have any other sepulcher than the heart and body where the root of this great love resided, and so for this reason, little by little, over a period of time, she drank these ashes mixed with wine until she had consumed them all. Nevertheless, she still wished to build a sepulcher to her husband's memory to serve forever as his memorial.[2]

---

1 Rembert Dodoens, *A Nievve Herball, or Historie of Plantes*, trans. Henry Lyte (London, 1578). Blanche Henrey discusses the relationship between Flemish and English frontispieces in *British Botanical and Horticultural Literature before 1800* (London: Oxford University Press, 1975), 32.

2 Christine de Pizan, *The Book of the City of Ladies*, trans. Earl Jeffrey Richards, (New York: Persea Books, 1982), 123.

The sorrow that surrounds her legend and her fame for being the first to make a mausoleum may give the flower Queen Artemisia holds in the frontispiece a wilting, funereal aspect. That the herb is "singular for womens disseases" (17)—in other texts called "women's griefs"—may inform its continued association with a female personage known for her sorrows. Though her widowhood has very little to do with her purported contributions to herbalism, we will soon see how her relationship to her husband comes to inform the etymological history of the herb.

The quartet of herbalist kings and queens of the frontispiece reappears in Lyte's dedication to Elizabeth I, drawing attention to their position as monarchs so "that thing may not iustly be thought unmeete to be offered unto a Prince";[3] Artemisia's name is listed last. The associations between the historical queen and the modern-day herb are then made more concrete in Gerard's address to his reader, in which he relates the long list of kings associated with herbal knowledge: "As for *Artemisia*, first called *πάρθενις* whether the title thereof sprang from 'ἀρτεμις, *Diana* hir selfe, or from the renowned Queene of Caria, which disclosed the vse thereof vnto posteritie, it suruiueth as a monument to reuiue the memories of them both for euer" (fol. 8v). Gerard cunningly combines both Artemisia's claims to fame, the mausoleum and the herb, in the word "monument." While the lists of monarchs who have a hand in herbal history in both Lyte and Gerard bear some relation to their source in Dodoens (and Dodoens' in Pliny), these references point to an extended continental tradition of invoking the figure of Artemisia as a precedent for sovereign contributions to herbal knowledge, a tradition on which all English texts draw.

The specific reference to Dodoens may also bring with it another aspect of the continental tradition, the precedent of a female royal patron. That is, Dodoens dedicates his 1554 Flemish text, which is the source of the frontispiece that portrays the forlorn Artemisia, to Mary of Austria, "Queen Dowager of Hungary and Bohemia" and "Regent and Governor" of the Netherlands.[4] Artemisia of Caria may be an even more direct prototype for the young Queen Mary, who never remarried after the tragic death of her husband. While Lyte may take his lead from the Flemish frontispiece, his inclusion of this list in his dedication may show a direct knowledge of Dodoens' Flemish text (the list is not included in the French prefatory materials) and thus a knowledge of its female patron. While Lyte translates the Flemish text through a French intermediary, he may have adapted the Dodoens' context—the governorship of Mary of Austria—directly to an English one—the reign of Elizabeth.

The processes of translation/selection at the root of the English herbal tradition are made apparent in interesting ways when it comes to statements about the naming of mugwort/artemisia. Turner's passage "Of Mugwurt" first appears in his 1551 *New Herball* and is reprinted as such in the 1568 edition. What is interesting here is the way in which Turner argues about the identification but not the name:

---

3 Lyte, "Dedicatory Epistle," in Dodoens, *A Nievve Herball*, *2r.

4 Rembert Dodoens, *Crŭijdeboeck* (Antwerp, 1554).

> The true artemisia is as lytle knowen nowe adayes as is ye true pontyke worm wode, & lesse, as I thinke. for this great mugwurt is such an artemisia, as our wormwood is absinthiū ponticum: that is, bastard, and not the true herbe. Dioscorides wryteth: y^{t} artemisia, for the most parte groweth about the see syde; and Pliny writeth: that it groweth no where elles, but in the see costes. This cōmon mugwurt of ours, groweth not at any see side, y^{t} euer I could se yet: for I coulde nether see it in these costes of england, nor germany, nor yet of Italy, but al waies in hedges, and amōg corne, far from ye see. . . . Wherefor this comō mugwurt can nether be artemisia of Dioscorides nor of Pliny. I found in an ylande beside venise, the very right artemisia . . . .master doctor Wendy, the kyngs Phisycyane can testifye of ye same, which dyd examyne ye herbe wyth me. Thys kynde may be called in Englysh sea mugwurt.[5]

The appearance of "doctor Wendy, the kyngs Phisycyane" as an authority reminds both the late sixteenth-century and the twenty-first-century reader of the context of the original composition under King Edward VI (d. 1553) and the contemporary noble reader of Turner's proximity to that authority. Significantly, for our purposes, this was written before England's first sovereign queen; this is not an Elizabethan entry.

The development after Turner seems to be in direct response to Dodoens. Lyte's rendition seems a straightforward translation of the French, a translation purportedly "supervised" by Dodoens himself.[6] Lyte's entry reads "Mugworte as *Plinie* saith, had this name of *Artemisia* Queen of *Halicarnassus* and wife of *Mausolus* king of Carie, who chose this herbe & gaue it her name" (in the original French: "qui choisit ceste herbe & luy imposa son nom"),[7] and this etymological history is then replicated almost exactly by Gerard, "Mugwoort is called in Latine *Artemisia*, which name it had of *Artemisia* Queen of Halicarnassus, and wife of noble *Mausolus* king of Caria, who adopted it for hir owne herbe."[8] There is no entry for "mugwort" or "artemisia" in *Paradisi in sole Paradisus Terrestris*, as it is not decorative and only medicinal, but in Parkinson's *Theatrum*, the entry says that artemisia "tooke the name of *Artemisia*, from *Artemisia* the wife of *Mausolus*, King of Caria."[9] The two sources for this history, Dodoens and Pliny, may account for the slight variations, but I would like to argue that after Lyte, with numerous sources in front of them, both Gerard and Parkinson made choices as to what they did and did not convey to their readers. That Lyte gives Artemisia a crown and a city as well as a marriage is determined by his Flemish/French source. Gerard's choice

---

5 William Turner, *A New Herball* (London, 1551), sigs. E1r–E1v.

6 Agnes Arber, *Herbals, their Origin and Evolution: A Chapter in the History of Botany, 1470–1670* (1912; reprint, Cambridge: Cambridge University Press, 1953), 82.

7 Lyte, trans., *A Nievve Herball*, 16, and Dodoens, *Histoires des Plantes*, trans. Charles de l'Écluse (Antwerp, 1557).

8 John Gerard, *The Herball or Generall Historie of Plantes* (London, 1597), 946.

9 John Parkinson, *Theatrum Botanicum, the Theater of Plantes* (London, 1640), 90.

in naming her "*Artemisia* Queen of Halicarnassus, and wife of noble *Mausolus* king of Caria," however, could be influenced by his Elizabethan context. Gerard's source is supposedly the Latin *Stirpium historiae pemptades sex* (1583), which puts the origins of the name in "*Artemisia Mausoli Cariæ Regis uxore, hanc sibi adoptante*."[10] The fact that the Latin makes no mention of Artemisia's position as queen but most definitely is the source for the variant phrase in Gerard's entry, "who adopted it for her owne herbe," shows that Gerard/Dr. Priest made a pointed selection in where and when he repeats Lyte's language. Parallel in difference is Parkinson's choice to ignore Gerard's and Lyte's translation and call up Pliny's designation of Artemisia as simply "the wife of Mausolus," a designation that takes away her sovereign rule after the death of her husband and perhaps makes a connection with Henrietta Maria, the queen-consort, who takes delight in flowers, rather than the so-depicted learned Elizabeth.[11]

This history shows how the political context may inform the developing discussion of herbs. Before the presence of a female sovereign, Turner's "artemisia" is interesting mainly for the issue of its location (or not) in England and its true identity. During the reign of Elizabeth, Artemisia's sovereign queenliness becomes an integral part of the herb's discussion. In a post-Elizabethan context, Artemisia loses her sovereign status and becomes queen-consort. All of which goes to prove that artemisia, by any other name, is (or is not) mugwort.

---

10 Rembert Dodoens, *Stirpivm Historiae Pemptades Sex* (Antwerp, 1583), 33.

11 Pliny the Elder, *Naturall History*, trans. W. H. S. Jones (Cambridge, Massachusetts: Harvard University Press, 1956), XXXV.73.

Appendix B
Female Owners of Herbal Texts[1]

My goal when starting this project—I admit somewhat arbitrarily—was to find twenty examples of early modern women's herbal ownership because I knew that extant copies numbering in the hundreds and limited time and resources would not allow for an exhaustive catalog of ownership. I did want, however, a substantial enough number of examples to be able to perform a comparative analysis. In the examples I give here, I have been able to estimate with reasonable (in some cases absolute) certainty that the ownership occurred before or soon after 1700. The majority of the attributions of ownership come by way of signatures I have found in the herbals themselves. The rest have been determined through other kinds of evidence: wills, inventories, commissioned artworks, autobiographical and literary manuscripts, household inventories, letters, and remedy books. The twenty-four examples I work with in the introduction and in Chapters 2 and 3 are as follows:

(1) Margaret Hoby's diary entries from 1599/1600;[2]
(2) Grace Mildmay's autobiography and medical papers;[3]
(3) Elizabeth Isham's 1648 Book Inventory lists "An Herball" at entry 41;[4]
(4) The left panel of "The Great Picture," likely by Jan van Belcamp and commissioned by Anne Clifford Herbert, Countess of Pembroke, in 1646,

---

[1] An earlier version of this list appears in the notes of Rebecca Laroche, "'To take in hand the practise of phisick': Early Modern Women's Signatures in Print Medical Texts," in *New Ways of Looking at Old Texts IV*, ed. Michael Denbo (Tempe, Arizona: Renaissance English Text Society, Spring 2009), 272–73.

[2] Joanna Moody, ed., Margaret Hoby, *The Private Life of an Elizabethan Lady: The Diary of Lady Margaret Hoby, 1599–1605* (Stroud, Gloucestershire: Sutton Publishing, 1998), references to the herbal are on pages 18, 29, and 58. See also Moody's note 18. n. 46, and Mary Ellen Lamb, "Margaret Hoby's Diary: Women's Reading Practices and the Gendering of the Reformation Subject," *Pilgrimage for Love: Essays in Early Modern Literature in Honor of Josephine A. Roberts*, ed. Sigrid King (Tempe, Arizona: Center for Medieval and Renaissance Studies, 1999), 90.

[3] Grace Mildmay, "Meditations," Northamptonshire Studies Collection, Northampton Central Library, part 1., fols. 10 and 46; see also Linda Pollock, *With Faith and Physic: The Life of a Tudor Gentlewoman, Lady Grace Mildmay, 1552–1620* (New York: St. Martin's Press, 1993), 26, 35.

[4] Elizabeth Isham, "Book Inventory," Northamptonshire Records Office, IC 4829.

depicts *The Epitome of Gerards Herball*, a volume that implies the presence of Gerard in the household;[5]

(5) Anne Southwell's miscellany contains a reference to books belonging to Anne and a list compiled by her husband, an item of which is "Gerard's Herball in folio";[6]

(6) Elizabeth Freke, whose manuscript at the British Library, Add. MS. 45718, contains "remedies abstracted from John Gerard's herbal";[7]

(7) Similarly, "A Booke of Hearbes & Receipts"(1627) with Elizabeth Bulckley's signature contains herbal entries distilled from Gerard's *Herball*;[8]

(8) Doreen Evenden Nagy cites Sara Gater's 1654 will as containing "Gerrards Herball";[9]

(9) Similarity in wording between a 1641 letter by Brilliana Harley and the relevant entries in the herbals make it likely that she consulted either Dodoens or Gerard (the latter having as a source the former) in her prescription of angelica for preventing the plague.[10]

The list of autographs (in order of discovery) is:

(10) Elizabeth Bagot's 1578 Dodoens *Nievve Herball* at the Yale Medical Historical Library, Herbal+;

(11) Anne Purefoy's 1629 *Paradisus Terrestris* (I included this volume though questionable in its genre because of the ways in which Parkinson refers to it as the first volume in a two-volume project), Folger STC 19300, Copy 1;

(12) "Ann Stoughton," in a Parkinson *Theatrum Botanicum*, information and copy of page provided for me by Jack Eckert, the Reference Librarian

---

5 Jan van Belcamp, "The Great Picture," c. 1646, Abbot Hall Art Gallery, Kendal, Cumbria. An online reproduction of the triptych can be found through the W. W. Norton site, http://www.wwnorton.com/college/english/nael/17thcentury/topic_1/illustrations/imclifford.htm (accessed February 25, 2009).

6 Anne Southwell, *The Southwell–Sibthorpe Commonplace Book: Folger MS. V.b. 198*, ed. Jean Klene (Tempe, Arizona: Medieval & Renaissance Texts & Studies, 1997), 99. The list is discussed as Southwell's in Heidi Brayman Hackel, *Reading Material in Early Modern England: Print, Gender, and Literacy* (Cambridge: Cambridge University Press, 2005), 216.

7 Elizabeth Freke, *The Remembrances of Elizabeth Freke*, ed. Raymond A. Anselment (Cambridge: University of Cambridge Press, 2001), 175.

8 Bulckley's manuscript can be viewed in *Women and Medicine: Remedy Books, 1533–1865, from the Wellcome Library for the Understanding and History of Medicine*, ed. Sara Pennell (Reading: Primary Source Microfilm, Thomas Gale, 2004), Reel 1.

9 Doreen Evenden Nagy, *Popular Medicine in Seventeenth-Century England* (Bowling Green, Ohio: Bowling Green State University Popular Press, 1988), 66.

10 Brilliana Harley, *Letters of the Lady Brilliana Harley, Wife of Sir Robert Harley, of Brampton Bryan, Knight of Bath*, ed. and intro. Thomas Taylor Lewis, A. M. (London: Camden Society, 1854), 129.

from the Countway Library of Medicine in Massachusetts who writes: "The Parkinson . . . has the ownership inscription [crossed out] of Ann Stoughton and, below that, one of Margret Massingberd."[11] Ann Stoughton's roman hand appears to be from the seventeenth-century, Countway Medicine, Rare Books f 1.Me.17;
(13) "Ann Loggin Her Boock," *Theatrum Botanicum*, Library of Congress, QK41 .P2 English Print Folio, copy 3;
(14) The wife of a John F. who died in 1672, according to his inscription and poem on the blank page after the front matter, *Theatrum Botanicum*, Library of Congress, QK41 .P2 Bitting Coll., copy 2;
(15) Signature of "Ann Parso[n]s" found in the New York Public Library's 1619 Dodoens, 3E3v, "Table of the Nature, Vertues, and Dangers," accompanies and, I argue, imitates an inscription "Sum liber Richard: Parsons: | Anno. 1628" from the second flyleaf recto (though possession per se is questionable, it does indicate herbal reading and "ownership" of another kind), NYPL *ZKC1410–6987;
(16) "Katherine Shirley | her booke" on the flyleaf of the Arizona State University Patten collection's 1629 *Paradisus Terrestris* accompanied by the Shirley coat of arms, Hayden Special Collection, SPEC PAT–138;
(17) "Ann Whithall is the owner of this booke," and "Anne Whitehall of Yildersley | her booke 1672," two separate ownership inscriptions from the 1578 Dodoens from the University of Pennsylvania, RBC Folio 580 D665 EL;
(18) "Jane Baker 1660," in a *Theatrum Botanicum* at the Academy of Natural Sciences, Philadelphia, QK41 .P23;[12]
(19) The inscription "Mary Ellys's booke bought of Sister Stacy" from the last page of a 1633 Gerard at the Moody Library at the University of Texas Medical Branch implies two female owners (counted here only as one entry), Rare Book Room 4TO;
(20) "Elizabeth Hamond," 1578 Dodoens, Houghton Library, f STC 6984;
(21) "Sarah Gibson," 1636 Gerard, Texas A&M Cushing Memorial Library, Rare Books, QK41 .G3 1636; date approximated through eighteenth-century provenance;
(22) "Mary Saltonstall 1674," written in the spiral flourish under the very large "Sr John Weld/Senio^r^ 1666," verso of dedication, 1629 Parkinson, Texas A&M, Cushing Memorial Library, Rare Books SB97 . P24 1629;
(23) "Elizabeth: Turner:" on the verso of the title page in the 1578 Dodoens at Huntington Library, Rare Books 60102 (reproduced in *Early English*

[11] Jack Eckert, e-mail message to author, January 4, 2006.

[12] I would also like to note here the beautiful later inscription, "Rachel Bolton her book A^{o}: D^{i}: 1767" also at the ANS in its 1636 Gerard.

Books Online);
(24) "Mary Chambers her book amen.1689" appears in the last page of the front matter of in the 1578 *Nievve Herball*, Linnaean Society Library, RF.578, Another copy.[13]

[13] My thanks to Karen Reeds for directing me to Mary Chambers's example. The remaining signatures that are yet to be seen or are more difficult to prove early modern: (25) Elena Sisti has informed me of the promising "Jane Wilcocks" in the Philadelphia Horticultural Society 1597 Gerard, e-mail to the author, July 5, 2007; (26) Karen Reeds has written me that she has seen the inscription "Jane Grace her booke 1666" in a 1586 Dodoens at the Bartram Garden Library in Philadelphia, e-mail to the author, November 18, 2008; (27) "Sarah Rodway her book March ye 16," William Turner's *A New Herbal* (London, 1551) at the Folger Shakespeare Library, Folger STC 24365.

At the time of writing this Appendix, I have considered around 140 examples of these volumes, making the occurrence of women's autographs just under one in ten. Of course, this number fluctuates with each library visited. Along with the librarians and archivists from the NYPL, Philadelphia Horticultural Society, Texas A&M, and UPenn collections listed above, all of whom took time to communicate with me via e-mail, I would like to thank Karen Kukil at Smith College, Eric Pomeroy at Bryn Mawr, Jill Gage at the Newberry, and Stacey Peeples at Pennsylvania Hospital, who looked at their collections for me.

Bibliography

Primary

Anon. *The Grete Herball*. London, 1626. STC 13176.

Anon. *A godly and holsom preseruatyue against disperacion at al times necessarye for the soule*. London, 1551.

Anon. *Here Begynneth a Good Booke of Medecines Called the Treasure of poore men*. London, [1560?]. STC 24206a.

Apuleius, Barbarus. *The Herbal of Pseudo-Apuleius: from the Ninth-Century Manuscript in the Abbey of Monte Cassino [Codex Casinensis 97]*. Described and annotated by F. W. T. Hunger. Leyden, 1935.

Bagot, Elizabeth. "Letter." Folger Manuscript L.a.48.

Becon, Thomas. *A pleasante newe Nosegaye*. London, 1542.

"A Booke of Hearbes & Receipts. 1627," Wellcome MS 169. *Women and Medicine: Remedy Books, 1533–1865, from the Wellcome Library for the Understanding and History of Medicine, London,* edited by Sara Pennell, Reel 1. Reading: Primary Source Microfilm, 2004.

Brackley, Elizabeth Cavendish, and Jane Cavendish. *The Concealed Fancies. Renaissance Drama by Women: Texts and Documents*. Edited by S. P. Cerasano and Marion Wynne-Davies, 127–54. Routledge: London, 1996.

Brasbridge, Thomas. *The Poore Mans levvel, that is to say, A Treatise of the Pestilence Unto the Which is Annexed a declaration of the vertues of the hearbs Carduus Benedictus and Angelica*. London: George Byshop, 1578. STC 3549.

Brunfels, Otto. *Herbarum Uiuae Eicones ad Naturae Imitationem, sum[m]a cum Diligentia & Artificio Effigiatae, una cum Effectibus Earundem, in Gratiam Ueteris Illius, & Iamiam Renascentis Herbariae Medicinae*. Argentorati: Apud Ioannem Schottu[m], 1532.

Bullein, William. *A newe boeke Entituled the Gouernement of Health: wherein is vttred manye notable Rules for mannes preseruacion, with sondry symples and other matters, no lesse fruitfull then profitable*. London, 1559. STC 4041.

——. *A Dialogve bothe pleasaunte and pietifull, wherein is a goodly regimente against the feuer Pestilence with a consolacion and comfort against death*. London, 1564. STC 4036.5.

Bush, Paul. *Certayne Gostly Medycynes to be Used to Eschew the Plage of Pestilence*. London, 1531.

Christine, De Pizan. *The Book of the City of Ladies*. Translated by Earl Jeffrey Richards. New York: Persea Books, 1982.

Culpeper, Nicholas. *The English Physitian or an Astrologo-physical Discourse of the Vulgar Herbs of this Nation*. London, 1652.

Day, Richard. *A Booke of Christian Prayers*. London, 1578. Facsimile, Walter J. Johnson, Inc. Theatrum Orbis Terrarum. Amsterdam, 1977.

Deacon, John. *Tobacco Tortvred, or, The Filthie Fvme of Tobacco Refined*. London, 1616. STC 6436.

Digby, Elizabeth. "Receipts of Elizabeth Digby." British Library MS Egerton 2197.

Dioscorides. *The Greek Herbal of Dioscorides*. Englished by John Goodyer, 1655. Edited by Robert T. Gunther. Oxford: Oxford University Press, 1934.

Dodoens, Rembert. *Crŭijdeboeck*. Antwerp, 1554.

——. *Histoires des Plantes*. Translated by Charles de l'Écluse. Anvers, 1557.

——. *A Nevv Herbal, or Historie of Plants*. Translated by Henry Lyte. London, 1619. STC 6987.

——. *A Nievve Herball, or Historie of Plantes*. Translated by Henry Lyte Esquyer. London, 1578. STC 6984.

——. *Stirpivm Historiae Pemptades Sex, Sive Libri XXX*. Antwerp, 1583.

Elizabeth I. *Collected Works*. Edited by Leah S. Marcus, Janel Mueller, and Mary Beth Rose. Chicago: University of Chicago Press, 2000.

Freke, Elizabeth. *The Remembrances of Elizabeth Freke, 1671–1714*. Edited by Raymond A. Anselment. Cambridge: Cambridge University Press for the Royal Historical Society, 2001.

Fuchs, Leonhart. *New Kreüterbuch*. Basell, 1543.

——. *The Great Herbal of Leonhart Fuchs: De Historia Stirpium Commentarii Insignes, 1542 (Notable Commentaries on the History of Plants)*. Edited and translated by Frederick G. Meyer, Emily Emmart Trueblood, and John L. Heller. Stanford: Stanford University Press, 1999.

B.G. [Bernard Garter]. *The Ioyfull Receyuing of the Queenes Most Excellent Maiestie into hir Highnesse Citie of Norwich*. London, 1578. STC 11627.

Gerard, John. *The Herball or Generall Historie of Plantes*. London, 1597. STC 11750.

——. *The Herball or Generall Historie of Plantes, Gathered by Iohn Gerard of London Master in Chirurgerie, Very much Enlarged and Amended by Thomas Iohnson, Citizen and Apothecarye*. London, 1633. STC 11751. Reprinted in 1636. STC 11752.

Gifford, George. *A Discourse of the subtill Practises of Deuilles by VVitches and Sorcerers*. London, 1587. STC 11852.

Goeurot, Jean. *The Regiment of lyfe, Wherunto is Added a Treatise of the Pestilence, with the Speciall Remedies (Experimented) for all Diseases, Griefes, Impediments, and Often Happening in Yong Children, newly Corrected and Enlarged by Thomas Phaire*. London, 1567. STC 11974.

Halkett, Anne. *The Memoirs of Anne, Lady Halkett and Ann, Lady Fanshawe*. Edited by John Loftis. Oxford: Clarendon Press, 1979.

Harley, Lady Brilliana. *Letters of the Lady Brilliana Harley, Wife of Sir Robert Harley, of Brampton Bryan, Knight of the Bath*. Edited and introduced by Thomas Taylor Lewis, A.M. London: Camden Society, 1854.

Hill, Thomas. *The Gardeners Labyrinth: containing a discourse of the gardeners life, in the yearly trauels to be bestovved on his plot of earth, for the vse of a garden*. London, 1577. STC 13485.

Hoby, Lady Margaret. *The Diary of Lady Margaret Hoby*. British Library Egerton MS 2614. In *Medieval and Early Modern Women*, Reel 9. Marlborough, Wiltshire: Adam Matthew Publishing, 2000–2004.

——. *Diary of Lady Margaret Hoby*. Edited by Dorothy M. Meads. London: George Routledge & Sons, 1930.

——. *The Private Life of an Elizabethan Lady: The Diary of Lady Margaret Hoby, 1599–1605*. Edited by Joanna Moody. Stroud, Gloucestershire: Sutton Publishing, 1998.

Holland, Henry. *A Treatise against VVitchcraft*. Cambridge, 1590. STC 13590.

Huntingdon, Elizabeth Hastings, Countess of. *Correspondence*. Huntington Library, Hastings Collection.

Hutchinson, Lucy. *Memoirs of the Life of Colonel Hutchinson*. Edited by James Sutherland. London: Oxford University Press, 1973.

Isham, Elizabeth. "Autobiography, ca. 1640s." Robert H. Taylor Collection. Princeton University Library RTC01 no. 62.

——. "Book Inventory." Northamptonshire Records Office IC 4829.

——. "Northamptonshire Diary." Northamptonshire Records Office IL 3365.

Knox, John. *A fort for the afflicted: VVherein are ministred many notable & excellent remedies against the stormes of tribulation*. London, 1580.

Langham, William. *The Garden of health, conteyning the sundry rare and hidden vertues and properties of all kindes of Simples and Plants*. London, 1597/8. STC 15195.

Lawson, William. *A New Orchard and Garden with The Country Housewifes Garden for hearbes of common vse*. London, 1618. STC 15329.

Markham, Gervase. *The English House-wife*. London, 1668. Reproduced in *Defining Gender, 1450–1910*. Marlborough, England: Adam Matthew Publications Ltd., 2005. http://www.gender.amdigital.co.uk/contents/image-viewing.aspx?imageid=5241 (accessed March 10, 2009).

Mattioli, Pietro Andrea. *Commentarii Secvndo Avcti, in Libros sex Pedacij Dioscoridis Anazarbei de Medica Materia*. Venice, 1560.

Meurier, Gabriel. *The Nosegay of Morall Philosophie*. Translated by Thomas Crew. London, 1580.

Mildmay, Lady Grace. "Meditations." Northamptonshire Studies Collection. Northampton Central Library. Parts 1 and 2.

——. "Medical Papers." Northamptonshire Record Office. W(A) misc. Vols. 32 and 33.

Moore, Philip. *The hope of Health wherein is conteined a goodlie Regimente of Life: As medicine, good diet, and the goodly vertues of Sonderie herbes*. London, 1565. STC 18059.5.

Moulton, Thomas. *The Myrrour or Glass of Healthe*. London, [1566]. STC 18224.

Parkinson, John. *Paradisi in Sole Paradisus Terrestris*. London, 1629. STC 19300.

——. *Theatrum Botanicum, the Theater of Plantes*. London, 1640. STC 19302.

Pena, Pierre, and Matthias de l'Obel. *Stirpium aduersaria noua*. London, 1570.

Perkins, William. *A Discourse of the Damned Art of Wtchcraft; so Farre Forth as it is Reuealed in the Scriptures, and Manifest by True Experience*. Cambridge, 1608. STC 19697.

Plat, Hugh. *The Iewell House of Art and Nature: Conteining diuers rare and profitable inuentions, together with sundry new experimentes in the art of husbandry, distillation, and moulding*. London, 1594. STC 19991.

Pliny the Elder. *Natural History, Vols. V–VII*. Translated by W. H. S. Jones. Cambridge, Massachusetts: Harvard University Press, 1956.

Ram, William. *Rams Little Dodeons* [sic], *a brief epitome of the new herbal or history of plants*. London, 1606. STC 6988.

Ramesey, William. *Thanasima Kai Dēlētēria Tractatus de Venenis, or, A Treatise of Poysons: Their sundry sorts, names, natures and virtues, with their severall symptomes, signes diagnosticks, prognosticks, and antidotes*. London, 1661.

Rid, Samuel. "The Art of Juggling or Legerdemain" (1612). In *Rogues, Vagabonds, & Sturdy Beggars*. Edited by Arthur F. Kinney, 261–91. Amherst: University of Massachusetts Press, 1990.

Shakespeare, William. *All's Well That Ends Well*. In *The Norton Shakespeare Based on the Oxford Edition*, edited by Stephen Greenblatt et al., 2175–2244. New York: W. W. Norton & Company, 1997.

——. *The Tragedy of Hamlet, Prince of Denmark*. In *The Norton Shakespeare*, 1659–1760.

——. *The Merry Wives of Windsor*. In *The Norton Shakespeare*, 1225–1292.

Shirley, Katherine. "Will." Public Records Office. Prob. 11/341. Fols. 12r–12v.

Southwell, Anne. *The Southwell–Sibthorpe Commonplace Book: Folger Ms. V.b. 198*. Edited by Jean Klene. Tempe, Arizona: Medieval & Renaissance Texts & Studies, 1997.

Spenser, Edmund. *The Faerie Queene*. Edited by Thomas P. Roche, Jr. London: Penguin, 1978.

Thynne, Maria. "Letters." In *Lay by Your Needles Ladies, Take the Pen: Writing Women in England, 1500–1700*, edited by Suzanne Trill, Kate Chedgzoy, and Melanie Osborne, 76–78. London: St. Martin's Press, 1997.

Turner, William. *Libellus de Re Herbaria, 1538, [and] The Names of Herbes, 1548*. Edited by William Thomas Stearn. London: Ray Society, 1965.

——. *A New Herball*. London, 1551. STC 24365.

——. *A new booke of spirituall Physik for dyuerse diseases of the nobilite and gentlemen of Englande*. Rome,1555.

——. *The Seconde Part of VVilliam Turners Herball*. Cologne, 1562.

——. *The first and seconde partes of the Herbal of William Turner Doctor in Phisick / lately ouersene / corrected and enlarged with the Thirde parte / lately gathered.* Cologne, [1568]. STC 24367.

Van Belcamp, Jan. "The Great Picture," c. 1646. Abbot Hall Art Gallery, Kendal, Cumbria.

Wheathill, Anne. *A handfull of holesome (though homelie) hearbs, gathered out of the goodlie garden of Gods most holie word; for the common benefit and comfortable exercise of all such as are deuoutlie disposed. Collected and dedicated to all religious Ladies, Gentlewomen, and others.* London, 1584. STC 25329.

Whitney, Isabella. *A Sweet Nosgay, or Pleasant Posy, 1573*. London, 1573. *Renaissance Women Online*, September, 1999. Women Writers Project. Brown University. http://textbase.wwp.brown.edu/WWO/php/rAll.php?doc=whitney.nosegay.html&num=00280 (accessed February 28, 2009).

Secondary

Achterberg, Jeanne. *Woman as Healer*. Boston: Shambhala Press, 1991.

Andersen, Jennifer, and Elizabeth Sauer, eds. *Books and Readers in Early Modern England: Material Studies*. Philadelphia: University of Pennsylvania Press, 2002.

Anderson, Frank J. *An Illustrated History of the Herbals*. New York: Columbia University Press, 1977.

Anselment, Raymond A. *The Realms of Apollo: Literature and Healing in Seventeenth-Century England.* Newark: University of Delaware Press, 1995.

Appelbaum, Robert. "Rhetoric and Epistemology in Early Printed Recipe Collections." *Journal of Early Modern Cultural Studies* 3.2 (2003): 1–35.

Apps, Lara, and Andrew Gow. *Male Witches in Early Modern Europe*. Manchester: Manchester University Press, 2003.

Arber, Agnes. *Herbals, their Origin and Evolution: A Chapter in the History of Botany, 1470–1670*. 1912. Reprint, Cambridge: Cambridge University Press, 1953.

Atkinson, Colin B., and Jo B. Atkinson. "Anne Wheathill's *A Handfull of Holesome (though Homelie) Hearbs* (1584): The First English Gentlewoman's Prayer Book." *The Sixteenth Century Journal* 27.3 (Fall 1996): 659–72.

Babcock, Robert G., et al. *A Book of Her Own: An Exhibition of Manuscripts and Printed Books in the Yale University Library that were Owned by Women Before 1700.* New Haven, Connecticut: Yale University Press, 2005.

Barrera, Antonio. "Local Herbs, Global Medicines: Commerce, Knowledge, and Commodities in Spanish Americas." In *Merchants and Marvels: Commerce,*

Science, and Art in Early Modern Europe, edited by Pamela H. Smith and Paula Findlen, 163–81. New York: Routledge, 2007.

Bayer, Penny. "Lady Margaret Clifford's Alchemical Receipt Book and the John Dee Circle." *AMBIX* 52.3 (November 2005): 271–84.

Beal, Peter. *In Praise of Scribes: Manuscripts and Their Makers in Seventeenth-Century England.* Oxford: Clarendon Press, 1998.

Beier, Lucinda McCray. *Sufferers and Healers: The Experience of Illness in Seventeenth-Century England.* London: Routledge & Kegan Paul, 1987.

Beilin, Elaine V. *Redeeming Eve: Women Writers of the English Renaissance.* Princeton: Princeton University Press, 1987.

Bell, Ilona. *Elizabethan Women and the Poetry of Courtship.* Cambridge: Cambridge University Press, 1998.

Berry, Boyd. "We are not all alyke nor of complexion one": Truism and Isabella Whitney's Multiple Readers." *Renaissance Papers* (2000): 13–23.

Brace, Patricia. "Isabella Whitney, *A Sweet Nosegay*." In *A Companion to Early Modern Women's Writing*, edited by Anita Pacheco, 97–109. Oxford: Blackwell Publishing, 2002.

——. "Teaching Class: Whitney's 'Wyll and Testament' and Nashe's 'Litany in Time of Plague.'" In *Teaching Tudor and Stuart Women Writers*, edited by Susanne Woods and Margaret Hannay, 279–82. New York: The Modern Language Assocation, 2000.

Brayman Hackel, Heidi. *Reading Material in Early Modern England: Print, Gender, and Literacy*. Cambridge: Cambridge University Press, 2005.

Brayman Hackel, Heidi, and Catherine E. Kelly, eds. *Reading Women: Literacy, Authorship and Culture in the Atlantic World, 1500–1800*. Philadelphia: University of Pennsylvania Press, 2008.

Bushnell, Rebecca. *Green Desire: Imagining Early Modern English Gardens*. Ithaca, New York: Cornell University Press, 2003.

Callery, Bernadette G. "Ancients, Moderns, and Reliable Friends: Stated Sources of Some English Herbals." *Journal of the Society for the Bibliography of Natural History*. 8.4 (1978): 435–44.

Chartier, Roger. *Cultural History: Between Practices and Representations*. Translated by Lydia G. Cochrane. Ithaca, New York: Cornell University Press, 1988.

Clarke, Elizabeth, and Erica Longfellow, dirs. *Constructing Elizabeth Isham*. http://www2.warwick.ac.uk/fac/arts/ren/projects/isham/ (accessed March 5, 2009).

Clarke, Elizabeth, and Martyn Bennett, dirs. *Perdita*. http://human.ntu.ac.uk/research/perdita/ (accessed July 27, 2005).

Clarkson, Leslie A. *Death, Disease, and Famine in Pre-Industrial England*. New York: St. Martin's Press, 1975.

Cody, Lisa Forman, ed. *Writings on Medicine*. Burlington, Vermont: Ashgate Publishing, 2002.

Cole, Mary Hill. *The Portable Queen: Elizabeth I and the Politics of Ceremony*. Amherst: University of Massachusetts Press, 1999.

Collinson, Patrick. "William Camden and the Anti-Myth of Elizabeth: Setting the Mould?" In *The Myth of Elizabeth*, edited by Susan Doran and Thomas S. Freeman, 79–98. Basingstoke: Palgrave Macmillan, 2003.

——. *The Birthpangs of Protestant England: Religious and Cultural Change in the Sixteenth and Seventeenth Centuries*. London: Macmillan Press, 1988.

Cooper, Alix. *Inventing the Indigenous: Local Knowledge and Natural History in Early Modern Europe*. Cambridge: Cambridge University Press, 2007.

Corbett, Marjorie. "The Engraved Title-page to John Gerarde's *herball or Generall Historie of Plantes*, 1597." *Journal of the Society for the Bibliography of Natural History* 8.3 (1977): 223–30.

Cressy, David. *Literacy and the Social Order: Reading and Writing in Tudor and Stuart England*. Cambridge: Cambridge University Press, 1980.

Defining Gender, 1450–1910. http://www.gender.amdigital.co.uk/index.aspx.

DeZur, Kathryn. "'Vaine Books' and Early Modern Women Readers." In *Reading and Literacy in the Middle Ages and Renaissance*, edited by Ian Frederick Moulton, 105–205. Turnhout, Belgium: Brepols, 2004.

DiMeo, Michelle. "The Draft of Elizabeth Isham's Medical Receipt Book." *Constructing Elizabeth Isham*. Edited by Elizabeth Clarke and Erica Longfellow. http://www2.warwick.ac.uk/fac/arts/ren/projects/isham/workshop/dimeo/ (accessed February 12, 2009).

DiMeo, Michelle and Rebecca Laroche, "Elizabeth Isham and Medicine." http://www2.warwick.ac.uk/fac/arts/ren/projects/isham/medicine/ (accessed February 12, 2009).

Donawerth, Jane. "Women's Poetry and the Tudor-Stuart System of Gift Exchange." In *Women, Writing, and the Reproduction of Culture in Tudor and Stuart Britain*, edited by Mary E. Burke, Jane Donawerth, Linda L. Dove, and Karen Nelson, 3–18. New York: Syracuse University Press, 2000.

Ehrenreich, Barbara, and Deirdre English. *Witches, Midwives, and Nurses: A History of Women Healers*. Old Westbury, New York: The Feminist Press, 1973.

Ellinghausen, Laurie. "Literary Property and the Single Woman in Isabella Whitney's *A Sweet Nosegay*." *Studies in English Literature* 45.1 (Winter 2005): 1–22.

Erler, Mary C. *Women, Reading, and Piety in Late Medieval England*. Cambridge: Cambridge University Press, 2002.

Ezell, Margaret J. M. *Social Authorship and the Advent of Print*. Baltimore: Johns Hopkins University Press, 1999.

——. *Writing Women's Literary History*. Baltimore: Johns Hopkins University Press, 1993.

Falco, Raphael. *Conceived Presences: Literary Genealogy in Renaissance England*. Amherst: University of Massachusetts Press, 1991.

Family Search. http://www.familysearch.org/ (accessed March 9, 2009).

Felch, Susan. "Ann Lock's Authorial Medicine." *Reformation* 2 (1997): 7–38.

Ferguson, Margaret. *Dido's Daughters: Literacy, Gender, and Empire in Early Modern England and France*. Chicago: University of Chicago Press, 2003.

Field, Catherine. "'Many Hands Hands': Writing the Self in Early Modern Women's Recipe Books." In *Genre and the Development of Women's Life Writing in Early Modern England*, edited by Michelle M. Dowd and Julie A. Eckerle, 49–63. Burlington, Vermont: Ashgate Press, 2007.

——. "'Sweet Practicer, Thy Physic I Will Try': Helena and her 'Good Receipt' in *All's Well, That Ends Well*." In *All's Well, That Ends Well: New Critical Essays*, edited by Gary Waller, 194–208. New York: Routledge, 2007.

Fissell, Mary. *Vernacular Bodies: The Politics of Reproduction in Early Modern England*. Oxford: Oxford University Press, 2004.

——. "The Marketplace of Print." In *Medicine and the Market in England and Its Colonies*, edited by Mark S. R. Jenner and Patrick Wallis, 108–32. Basingstoke, Hampshire: Palgrave Macmillan, 2007.

——. *Patients, Power, and the Poor in Eighteenth-Century Bristol*. Cambridge: Cambridge University Press, 1991.

Frye, Susan. "Sewing Connections: Elizabeth Tudor, Mary Stuart, Elizabeth Talbot, and Seventeenth-Century Anonymous Needleworkers." In *Maids and Mistresses, Cousins and Queens: Women Alliances in Early Modern England*. edited by Susan Frye and Karen Robertson, 165–82. New York: Oxford University Press, 1999.

Frye, Susan, and Karen Robertson, eds. *Maids and Mistresses, Cousins and Queens: Women Alliances in Early Modern England*. New York: Oxford University Press, 1999.

Furdell, Elizabeth Lane. *Publishing and Medicine in Early Modern England*. Rochester, New York: University of Rochester Press, 2002.

Genette, Gérard. *Paratexts: Thresholds of Interpretation*. Translated by Jane E. Lewin. Cambridge: Cambridge University Press, 1997.

Gettings, Fred. *Dictionary of Occult and Alchemical Sigils*. London: Routledge, 1981.

Gillespie, Katharine. *Domesticity and Dissent in the Seventeenth Century: English Women Writers and the Public Sphere*. Cambridge: Cambridge University Press, 2004.

Gim, Lisa. "'Faire *Eliza's* Chaine': Two Female Writers' Literary Links to Queen Elizabeth I," *Maids and Mistresses, Cousins and Queens: Women's Alliances in Early Modern England*, edited by Susan Frye and Karen Robertson, 183–98. New York: Oxford University Press, 1999.

Givens, Jean A., Karen M. Reeds, and Alain Touwaide, eds. *Visualizing Medieval Medicine, 1200–1500*. Burlington, Vermont: Ashgate Publishing, 2006.

Glenn, Cheryl. *Rhetoric Retold: Regendering the Tradition from Antiquity through the Renaissance*. Carbondale and Edwardsville: Southern Illinois University Press, 1997.

Gough, Melinda. "'Not as Myself': The Queen's Voice in *Tempe Restored.*" *Modern Philology* 101.1 (August 2003): 48–67.

Green, Monica H. *Making Women's Medicine Masculine: The Rise of Male Authority in Pre-Modern Gynaecology*. Oxford: Oxford University Press, 2008.

Griffiths, Jeremy, ed. *The Tollemache Book of Secrets: A Descriptive Index and Complete Facsimile with an Introduction and Transcription Together with Catherine Tollemache's Receipts of Pastery, Confectionary & c*, completed by A. S. G. Edwards. London: Roxburghe Club, 2001.

Hackett, Helen. *Virgin Mother, Maiden Queen: Elizabeth I and the Cult of the Virgin Mary*. New York: St. Martin's Press, 1995.

Hageman, Elizabeth H., and Katherine Conway, eds. *Resurrecting Elizabeth I in Seventeenth-Century England.* Madison, New Jersey: Fairleigh Dickinson University Press, 2007.

Harkness, Deborah E. *The Jewel House: Elizabethan London and the Scientific Revolution*. New Haven, Connecticut: Yale University Press, 2007.

Harris, Jonathan Gil. *Foreign Bodies and the Body Politic: Discourses of Social Pathology in Early Modern England.* Cambridge: Cambridge University Press, 1998.

Hellwarth, Jennifer Wynne. "'Be unto me as a precious ointment': Lady Grace Mildmay, Sixteenth-Century Female Practitioner." *Dynamis* 19 (1999): 95–117.

Henrey, Blanche. *British Botanical and Horticultural Literature before 1800: Comprising a History and Bibliography of Botanical and Horticultural Books Printed in England, Scotland, and Ireland from the Earliest Times until 1800.* Volume 1. London: Oxford University Press, 1975.

Hill, Christopher. "Censorship and English Literature." In *The Collected Essays of Christopher Hill, Volume I: Writing and Revolution in 17th Century England,* 32–71. Amherst: University of Massachusetts Press, 1985.

——. "The Medical Profession and Its Radical Critics." In *Change and Continuity in Seventeenth-Century England*, 157–77. Cambridge, Massachusetts: Harvard University Press, 1975.

Hobby, Elaine. *Virtue of Necessity: English Women's Writing, 1649–88*. Ann Arbor: University of Michigan Press, 1989.

Hunter, Lynette. "Women and Domestic Medicine: Lady Experimenters, 1570–1620." In *Women, Science and Medicine 1500–1700: Mothers and Sisters of the Royal Society*, edited by Lynette Hunter and Sarah Hutton, 89–107. Stroud, Gloucestershire: Sutton Publishing, 1997.

Hurd-Mead, Kate Campbell. *A History of Women in Medicine, from the Earliest Times to the Beginning of the Nineteenth Century.* Haddam, Connecticut: The Haddam Press, 1938.

Jackson, Benjamin Daydon. "A Life of William Turner, 1877." Introductory Matter to William Turner's *Libellus de Re Herbaria, 1538* and *The Names of Herbes, 1548*. London: Ray Society, 1965.

Janowitz, Henry D. "Helena's Medicine in *All's Well that Ends Well*: Is it Paracelsian or Hermetical in Origin?" *Cauda Pavonis: Studies in Hermeticism* 20.1 (Spring 2001): 20–22.

Jeffers, Robert H. *The Friends of John Gerard (1545–1612): Surgeon and Botanist.* Falls Village, Connecticut: The Herb Grower Press, 1967.

Jenner, Mark S. R., and Patrick Wallis, eds. *Medicine and the Market in England and Its Colonies, c. 1450–c. 1850*. Basingstoke: Palgrave Macmillan, 2007.

Johns, Adrian. *The Nature of the Book: Print and Knowledge in the Making*. Chicago: University of Chicago Press, 1998.

Johnson, Francis. "Notes on English Retail Book-Prices, 1550–1640." *The Library* 5.5 (1950–51): 83–112.

Jones, Ann Rosalind, *The Currency of Eros: Women's Love Lyric in Europe, 1540–1620*. Bloomington: Indiana University Press, 1990.

Jones, Ann Rosalind and Peter Stallybrass. "The Politics of *Astrophil and Stella*." *Studies in English Literature, 1500–1900* 24.1 (1984): 53–68.

Keiser, George R. "Reconstructing Robert Thornton's Herbal." *Medium Aevum* 65.1 (1996): 35–53.

——. "Through a Fourteenth-Century Gardener's Eyes: Henry Daniel's Herbal." *Chaucer Review: A Journal of Medieval Studies and Literary Criticism* 31.1 (1996): 58–75.

Kerwin, William. *Beyond the Body: The Boundaries of Medicine and English Renaissance Drama.* Amherst: University of Massachusetts Press, 2005.

Knight, Leah. *Of Books and Botany in Early Modern England.* Burlington, Vermont: Ashgate Publishing, 2009.

Kors, Alan Charles, and Edward Peters, eds. *Witchcraft in Europe, 400–1700: A Documentary History*. Second Edition, revised by Edward Peters. Philadelphia: University of Pennsylvania Press, 2001.

Lamb, Mary Ellen. "Constructions of Women Readers." In *Teaching Tudor and Stuart Women Writers*, edited by Susanne Woods and Margaret P. Hannay, 23–34. New York: Modern Language Association of America, 2000.

Lamb, Mary Ellen. "Isabella Whitney and the Travails of Service." Paper presented at the meeting of the Renaissance Society of America, Miami, Florida. March 24, 2007.

——. "Margaret Hoby's Diary: Women's Reading Practices and the Gendering of the Reformation Subject." In *Pilgrimage for Love: Essays in Early Modern Literature in Honor of Josephine A. Roberts*, edited by Sigrid King, 63–94. Tempe, Arizona: Center for Medieval and Renaissance Studies, 1999.

Laroche, Rebecca. "'To take in hand the practise of phisick': Early Modern Women's Signatures in Print Medical Texts." In *New Ways of Looking at Old Texts IV*, edited by Michael Denbo, 269–78. Tempe, Arizona: Renaissance English Text Society, 2009.

——. "The Burton Herbal." *Notes and Queries* 252.4 (December 2007): 393–95.

——. "Elizabeth Bagot's Herbal." *Yale University Library Gazette*. 82.1–2 (October 2006): 21–26.

——. “Gendering Hands, Gendering Business: A Letter from Elizabeth Bagot. http://www.folger.edu/html/folger_institute/mm/EssayRL.html (accessed March 5, 2009).

——. “Catherine Tollemache’s Library.” *Notes and Queries* 251.2 (June 2006): 157–58.

——. “Pamphilia Across a Crowded Room: Mary Wroth’s Entry into the Canon.” *Genre* 30.4 (Winter 1997): 267–88.

Leong, Elaine, ed. *Receipt Books, c.1575–1800 from the Folger Shakespeare Library*. Marlborough,Wiltshire: Adam Matthew Publications, Ltd., 2006.

——. “Medical Recipe Collections in Seventeenth-Century England: Knowledge, Gender and Text.” Ph.D. Thesis, University of Oxford, 2005/06.

Leong, Elaine, and Sara Pennell, “Recipe Collections and the Currency of Medical Knowledge in the Early Modern ‘Medical Marketplace.’” In *Medicine and the Market in England and Its Colonies, c. 1450–c.1850*, edited by Mark S. R. Jenner and Patrick Wallis, 132–53. (Basingstoke, Hampshire: Palgrave Macmillan, 2007).

Lewalski, Barbara. *Writing Women in Jacobean England*. Cambridge, Massachusetts: Harvard University Press, 1993.

Lysons, Daniel. *The Environs of London: Being an Historical Account of the Towns, Villages, and Hamlets, within Twelve Miles of that Capital*, Vols. III and IV. London, 1795 and 1796.

MacFarlane, Alan. *Witchcraft in Tudor and Stuart England: A Regional and Comparative Study*. New York: Harper and Row Publishers, 1970.

MacKeon, Michael. *The Secret History of Domesticity: Public, Private, and the Division of Knowledge*. Baltimore: Johns Hopkins University Press, 2005.

Maclean, Ian. *The Renaissance Notion of Woman: A Study in the Fortunes of Scholasticism and Medical Science in European Intellectual Life*. Cambridge: Cambridge University Press, 1980.

Magnusson, Lynne. *Shakespeare and Social Dialogue: Dramatic Language and Elizabethan Letters*. Cambridge: Cambridge University Press, 1999.

Marotti, Arthur. “‘Love is not love’: Elizabethan Sonnet Sequences and the Social Order.” *English Literary History* 49.2 (1982): 396–428.

Martin, Randall. “The Autobiography of Grace, Lady Mildmay.” *Renaissance and Reformation* 18.1 (1994): 33–81.

McBride, Kari Boyd. “Contextual Materials for ‘A Chaine of Pearl’ by Diana Primrose.” Introductions to Works, *Renaissance Women Online*. Women Writers Project, Brown University. http://textbase.wwp.brown.edu/WWO/php/rInt.php?doc=rInt.00272.html (accessed March 2, 2009).

McGrath, Lynette. *Subjectivity and Women’s Poetry in Early Modern England*. Aldershot: Ashgate Publishing, 2002.

McKitterick, David. “Women and their Books in Seventeenth-Century England.” *The Library* 1.4 (December 2000): 359–80.

McNeill, Fiona. *Poor Women in Shakespeare*. Cambridge: Cambridge University Press, 2007.

Mirabella, Bella. "'Quacking Delilahs': Female Mountebanks in Early Modern England and Italy." In *Women Players in England, 1500–1650: Beyond the All-Male Stage*, edited by Pamela Allen Brown and Peter Parolin, 89–105. Burlington, Vermont: Ashgate Publishing, 2005.

Morgan, Paul. "Frances Wolfreston and "Hor Bouks': A Seventeenth-Century Woman Book-Collector." *The Library* 6.2 (1989): 197–219.

Mortimer, Ian. "The Rural Medical Marketplace in Southern England, c. 1570–1720." In *Medicine and the Market in England and Its Colonies, c. 1450–1850*." Edited by Mark S. R. Jenner and Patrick Wallis, 69–87.Basingstoke, Hampshire: Palgrave Macmillan, 2007.

Moss, Stephanie, and Kaara L. Peterson, eds. *Disease, Diagnosis, and Cure on the Early Modern Stage*. Burlington, Vermont: Ashgate, 2004.

Munkhoff, Richelle. "Searchers of the Dead: Authority, Marginality, and the Interpretation of Plague in England, 1574-1665." *Gender & History* 11.1 (April 1999): 1–29.

Munroe, Jennifer. *Gender and the Garden in Early Modern English Literature*. Burlington, Vermont: Ashgate Publishing, 2008.

Nagy, Doreen Evenden. *Popular Medicine in Seventeenth-Century England*. Bowling Green, Ohio: Bowling Green State University Popular Press, 1988.

Orgel, Stephen. "Marginal Maternity: Reading Lady Anne Clifford's *A Mirror for Magistrates*." In *Printing and Parenting in Early Modern England*, edited by Douglas A. Brooks, 267–89. Burlington, Vermont: Ashgate Publishing, 2005.

Orlin, Lena Cowen. "Chronicles of Private Life." In *The Cambridge Companion to English Literature, 1500–1600*, edited by Arthur Kinney, 241–64. Cambridge: Cambridge University Press, 2000.

——. "Gertrude's Closet." *Shakespeare Jahrbuch* 134 (1998): 44–67.

——. *Private Matters and Public Culture in Post-Reformation England*. Ithaca, New York: Cornell University Press, 1994.

Oxford Dictionary of National Biography, Online Version. Oxford: Oxford University Press, 2004–06. http://www.oxforddnb.com (accessed March 5, 2009).

The Oxford English Dictionary, 2nd ed. *OED Online*. Oxford: Oxford University Press, 1989. http://dictionary.oed.com (accessed March 5, 2009).

Painter, Robert, and Brian Parker. "Ophelia's Flowers Again." *Notes and Queries* 239.1 (March 1994): 42–43.

Panofsky, Richard J., ed. The Floures of Philosophie *(1572) by Sir Hugh Plat and* A Sweet Nosgay *(1573) and* The Copy of a Letter *(1567) by Isabella Whitney*. Delmar, New York: Scholar's Facsimiles and Reprints, 1982.

Parkinson, Ann. *Nature's Alchemist: John Parkinson, Herbalist to Charles I*. London: Frances Lincoln Limited, 2007.

Peck, Linda Levy. *Consuming Splendor: Society and Culture in Seventeenth-Century England*. Cambridge: Cambridge University Press, 2005.

——. *The Mental World of the Jacobean Court*. Cambridge: Cambridge University Press, 1991.

Pelling, Margaret, and Charles Webster, "Medical Practitioners," *Health, Medicine and Mortality in the Sixteenth Century*, 165–236. Cambridge: Cambridge University Press, 1979.

Pelling, Margaret, with Frances White. *Medical Conflicts in Early Modern London: Patronage, Physicians, and Irregular Practitioners, 1550–1640*. Oxford: Clarendon Press, 2003.

——. "Trade or Profession? Medical Practice in Early Modern England." In *The Common Lot: Sickness, Medical Occupations and the Urban Poor in Early Modern England*, 230–58. Harlow, Essex: Longman, 1998.

——."Compromised by Gender: the Role of the Male Medical Practitioner in Early Modern England." In *The Task of Healing: Medicine, Religion and Gender in England and the Netherlands, 1450–1800*, edited by Hilary Marland and Margaret Pelling, 101–33. Rotterdam: Erasmus Publishing, 1996.

Pembroke, Anne Clifford Herbert, Countess of. *The Memoir of 1603 and The Diary of 1616–1619*. Edited by Katherine O. Acheson. Peterborough, Ontario: Broadview Editions, 2007.

Pennell, Sara. "Perfecting Practice? Women, Manuscript Recipes, and Knowledge in Early Modern England." In *Early Modern Women's Manuscript Writing*, edited by Victoria E. Burke and Jonathan Gibson, 237–58. Aldershot, Hampshire: Ashgate Publishing, 2004.

Pennell, Sara, ed. *Women and Medicine: Remedy Books, 1533–1865, from the Wellcome Library for the Understanding and History of Medicine*. Reading: Primary Source Microfilm, 2004.

Peters, Julie Stone. *Theatre of the Book, 1480–1880: Print, Text, and Performance in Europe*. Oxford: Oxford University Press, 2000.

Pettigrew, Todd H. J. *Shakespeare and the Practice of Physic: Medical Narratives on the Early Modern Stage*. Newark: University of Delaware Press, 2007.

Phillippy, Patricia. "The Maid's Lawful Liberty: Service, the Household, and 'Mother B' in Isabella Whitney's *A Sweet Nosegay*." *Modern Philology* 95.4 (1998): 439–62.

Pollard, Tanya. *Drugs and Theater in Early Modern England*. Oxford: Oxford University Press, 2005.

Pollock, Linda. *With Faith and Physic: The Life of a Tudor Gentlewoman, Lady Grace Mildmay, 1552–1620*. New York: St. Martin's Press, 1993.

Porter, Roy. *Health for Sale: Quackery in England 1660–1850*. Manchester: Manchester University Press, 1989.

Porter, Roy, ed. *Patients and Practitioners: Lay Perceptions of Medicine in Pre-Industrial Society*. Cambridge: Cambridge University Press, 1985.

Prest, John. *Garden of Eden: The Botanic Garden and the Recreation of Paradise*. New Haven, Connecticut: Yale University Press, 1981.

Purkiss, Diane. *The Witch in History: Early Modern and Twentieth-Century Representations*. New York: Routledge, 1996.

Rackin, Phyllis. *Shakespeare and Women*. Oxford: Oxford University Press, 2005.

Rawcliffe, Carole. *Medicine and Society in Later Medieval England*. Stroud, Gloucestershire: Sutton Publishing, 1995.

Reeds, Karen. *Botany in Medieval and Renaissance Universities*. New York: Garland Publishing, 1991.

Reeves, Eileen. "Old Wives Tales and the New World System." *Configurations* 7.3 (1999): 301–54.

Riddle, John M. *Eve's Herbs: A History of Contraception and Abortion in the West*. Cambridge, Massachusetts: Harvard University Press, 1997.

Robbins, Rossell Hope. "Medical Manuscripts in English." *Speculum* 45.3 (July 1970): 393–415.

Roberts, Sasha. *Reading Shakespeare's Poems in Early Modern England*. Basingstoke, Hampshire: Palgrave Macmillan, 2003.

Rohde, Eleanour Sinclair. *The Old English Herbals*. 1922. Reprint, New York: Dover Publications, Inc., 1971.

S. E. B. "An Elizabethan Herbal." *More Books: A Bulletin of the Boston Public Library* 25 (1940): 245–46.

Schiebinger, Londa. *Plants and Empire: Colonial Bioprospecting in the Atlantic World*. Cambridge, Massachusetts: Harvard University Press, 2004.

——. *Nature's Body: Gender in the Making of Modern Science*. Boston: Beacon Press, 1993.

——. *The Mind Has No Sex? Women in the Origins of Modern Science*. Cambridge, Massachusetts: Harvard University Press, 1989.

Schurink, Fred. "An Elizabethan Grammar School Exercise Book." *Bodleian Library Record* 18.2 (October 2003): 174–96.

Sedgwick, Eve Kosofsky. *Between Men: English Literature and Male Homosocial Desire*. New York: Columbia University Press, 1985.

Seelig, Sharon. *Autobiography and Gender in Early Modern Literature: Reading Women's Lives, 1600–1680*. Cambridge: Cambridge University Press, 2006.

Shapin, Steven. *A Social History of Truth: Civility and Science in Seventeenth-Century England.* Chicago: The University of Chicago Press, 1994.

Shapiro, James. *Rival Playwrights, Marlowe, Jonson, Shakespeare*. New York: Columbia University Press, 1991.

Sherman, William. *Used Books: Marking Readers in Renaissance England*. Philadelphia: University of Pennsylvania Press, 2008.

——. "What Did Renaissance Readers Write in Their Books?" In *Books and Readers in Early Modern England: Material Studies*, edited by Jennifer Andersen and Elizabeth Sauer, 119–37. Philadelphia: University of Pennsylvania Press, 2002.

Shirley, Evelyn Philip. *Stemmata Shirleiana; or the Annals of the Shirley Family, Lords of Nether Etindon in the County of Warwick, and of Shirley in the County of Derby.* London: Nichols and Sons, 1873.

Shrank, Cathy. *Writing the Nation in Reformation England, 1530–1580*. Oxford: Oxford University Press, 2004.

Shteir, Ann B. *Cultivating Women, Cultivating Science*. Baltimore: Johns Hopkins University Press, 1996.

Siraisi, Nancy G. *Medieval & Early Renaissance Medicine: An Introduction to Knowledge and Practice*. Chicago: The University of Chicago Press, 1990.

Slack, Paul. "Mirrors of Health and Treasures of Poor Men: The Uses of Vernacular Medical Literature of Tudor England." In *Health, Medicine, and Mortality in the Sixteenth Century*, edited by Charles Webster, 237–73. Cambridge: Cambridge University Press, 1979.

Smith, Pamela H., and Paula Findlen, eds. *Merchants and Marvels: Commerce, Science, and Art in Early Modern Europe*. New York: Routledge, 2002.

Smuts, R. Malcolm. *Court Culture and the Origins of a Royalist Tradition in Early Stuart England*. Philadelphia: University of Pennsylvania Press, 1987.

Snook, Edith. *Women, Reading, and the Cultural Politics of Early Modern England*. Aldershot, Hampshire: Ashgate Publishing, 2005.

Spence, Richard. *Lady Anne Clifford, Countess of Pembroke, Dorset and Montgomery (1590–1676)*. Stroud, Gloucestershire: Sutton Publishing, 1997.

Spufford, Margaret. *Small Books and Pleasant Histories: Popular Fiction and Its Readership in Seventeenth-Century England*. Athens: The University of Georgia Press, 1981.

Stannard, Jerry. "The Plant Called Moly." In *Herbs and Herbalism in the Middle Ages and Renaissance*, edited by Katherine E. Stannard and Richard Kay, 254–307. Aldershot, Hampshire: Ashgate Variorum, 1999.

Steen, Sara Jayne. "Contextual Materials for *A Sweet Nosgay*," Introductions to Works, *Renaissance Women Online*. September 1999, Women Writers Project. Brown University.http://textbase.wwp.brown.edu/WWO/php/rInt.php?doc=rInt.00280.html&LT (accessed March 2, 2009).

Stensgaard, Richard K. "*All's Well That Ends Well* and the Galenico-Paracelsian Controversy." *Renaissance Quarterly* 25 (1972): 173–88.

Stephens, Isaac. "The Courtship and Singlehood of Elizabeth Isham, 1630–1634." *The Historical Journal* 51.1 (2008): 1–25.

Stephens, Isaac, ed. "The Autobiography of Elizabeth Isham." http://history.ucr.edu/people/grad_students/stephens/TheAutobiography.pdf (accessed March 11, 2009).

Stevenson, Jane. *Women Latin Poets: Language, Gender, and Authority, from Antiquity to the Eighteenth Century*. Oxford: Oxford University Press, 2005.

Stine, Jennifer. "Opening Closets: The Discovery of Household Medicine in Early Modern England." Ph.D. diss., Stanford University, 1996.

Strong, Roy. *The Renaissance Garden in England*. London: Thames and Hudson, 1979.

Tannenbaum, Rebecca. *The Healer's Calling: Women and Medicine in Early New England*. Ithaca, New York: Cornell University Press, 2002.

University of Oxford. *Alumni Oxonienses*, Vol. 1, 1500–1714. Nendeln/Liechtenstein: Kraus, 1968.

Walker, Kim. *Women Writers of the English Renaissance*. New York: Twayne Publishers, 1996.

Wall, Wendy. *Staging Domesticity: Household Work and English Identity in Early Modern Drama*. Cambridge: Cambridge University Press, 2002.

——. "Authorship and the Material Conditions of Writing." *The Cambridge Companion to English Literature, 1500–1600*. Edited by Arthur F. Kinney, 64–89. Cambridge: Cambridge University Press, 2000.

——. *The Imprint of Gender: Authorship and Publication in the English Renaissance*. Ithaca, New York: Cornell University Press, 1993.

Warren, Nancy Bradley. "Tudor Religious Cultures in Practice: The Piety and Politics of Grace Mildmay and Her Circle." *Literature Compass* 3.5 (September 2006): 1011–43.

Watkins, John. *Representing Elizabeth in Stuart England: Literature, History, and Sovereignty.* Cambridge: Cambridge University Press, 2002.

Watt, Tessa. *Cheap Print and Popular Piety, 1550–1640*. Cambridge: Cambridge University Press, 1991.

Wear, Andrew. *Knowledge and Practice in English Medicine, 1550–1680*. Cambridge: Cambridge University Press, 2000.

Webster, Charles, ed. *Health, Medicine, and Mortality in the Sixteenth Century*. Cambridge: Cambridge University Press, 1979.

Williamson, George C. *Lady Anne Clifford, Countess of Dorset, Pembroke & Montgomery, 1590–1676: Her Life, Letters and Work*. East Ardsley, Yorkshire: S. R. Publishers, 1967.

Wilson, Elkin Calhoun. *England's Eliza*. Cambridge, Massachusetts: Harvard University Press, 1939.

Women Writers Online. http://textbase.wwp.brown.edu/WWO/ (accessed March 11, 2009).

Woodward, Marcus. *Gerard's Herball: The Essence thereof Distilled by Marcus Woodward*. London: Gerald Howe, 1927.

Index

References to illustrations are in **bold**